Conquering Hepatitis C
and
Surviving Treatment

AN ESSENTIAL GUIDE
THROUGH EVERY STEP OF THE
HCV TREATMENT PROCESS
COMPANION WEBSITE: WWW.HCVSHARE.ORG

Tim Duncan - Cate Olivolo, MSN, FNP-C

Dedication

This book is dedicated to the many individuals who have undergone treatment and fought their best fight towards beating infection of the Hepatitis C Virus (HCV). While some clear the virus with little problem during treatment, there are those who need to go through extended treatment periods. Sometimes it may be necessary to take extra medications in order to continue on the standard medications. These efforts are nothing short of heroic.

Special thanks and gratitude needs to be given to those who wrote their personal testimony of their HCV history and their treatment experiences. No other sense of their feelings and emotions can be better obtained than by reading these stories; their selflessness to share their personal stories to help others who are infected with HCV commands very special recognition for these very special individuals. One of their stories is included at the beginning of each major section throughout the book.

We also want to recognize all the caregivers and families of those who have undergone treatment. Their loving aid and support makes the treatment process much more bearable and possibly prevents some from discontinuing treatment early. Finally, we want to send our thoughts and prayers to those who have succumbed to the more serious effects of this silent killer, Hepatitis C, and to their friends and families; there are those who have fought tremendously heroic fights for years to only lose their battle in the end.

Our sincerest hope is that by reading and following the suggestions in this guide through the treatment process, there will be many who will be able to tip the scales of chance in their favor and achieve a successful treatment outcome by eliminating the Hepatitis C virus from their body. It is a challenging thing to embark upon HCV eradication, but we think this guide through the treatment process will help enable you to maximize your chances of conquering Hepatitis C and survive the rigors of treatment during the process.

Foreword

I have been advising and treating people who have Hepatitis C infection since the mid 90's when treatment had only a 25% chance of curing the infection and thereby preventing cirrhosis, liver failure, and liver cancer. These lethal complications occur after the virus has infected the liver for decades, often not causing any symptoms, but attracting the attention of the immune system which tries its best to kill the virus. It will be successful and cure the infection 15% of the time, more frequently in younger patients, and rarely if you are infected over the age of 40.

2010 therapy can be expected to cure Hep C infection in 45% of genotype 1 and 80% of type 2 and 3. In 2011 we are expecting the arrival of protease and polymerase inhibitors, which increase the cure rate for genotype 1 patients to 80%. That is the good news.

The bad news is that the Hepatitis C virus, which has been smoldering in the liver for decades, will often have caused so much liver damage, that in the next 10 years we will see many more people develop liver failure and liver cancer than we have ever seen before. If we can eradicate the Hepatitis C infection before this happens, we can prevent many deaths from the complications of Hepatitis C.

The key to an SVR, or to a cure of Hep C infection, is to take the full dose of the medicines prescribed for therapy.

Pegylated Interferon, Ribavirin, and especially the new drugs must be taken on schedule so that the virus does not develop resistance to treatment. If a person misses even a few doses of the protease inhibitor, resistance may occur and treatment will fail.

This book, *Conquering Hepatitis C and Surviving Treatment*, will help both patients and health care providers get through the many side effects of therapy and result in the best chance for a successful outcome. As Everett Koop said when he was Surgeon General, "If you don't take your medicine, it is unlikely to work."

This book will empower patients by suggesting different strategies they can use to cope with side effects. The stories told by patients on therapy will inspire all of us and remind us of how much treatment affects daily life. More Hep C patients will die of complications of their infection in the upcoming decade (2010-2020) than have ever died before.

Every patient with Hepatitis C needs to be diagnosed, and their health care provider needs to discuss the pros and cons of treatment. If the promise of curing 80% of Hepatitis C infections with the addition of new drugs is borne out, we should be able to save many lives with therapy.

This book will enable patients to complete their treatment and fight their best fight against the potentially lethal Hepatitis C infection.

PAUL SCHLEINITZ MD, APRIL 20, 2010, MEDFORD, OREGON

1

Introduction

To know a thing is to have power over it. Treatment is an individual choice. If you are reading this, you've either made the decision to treat the Hepatitis virus or have been given the option. Either way, we hope this guide gives you support for your decision and provides a resource to answer your questions regarding the treatment process. We also encourage you to visit and check out our companion online support website; there you will find people who are undergoing HCV treatment that come together online to support each other during the treatment process. There are also many available resources for easy reference included there. It is located at www.hcvshare.org.

We, the authors, were previously diagnosed with Chronic HCV and experienced treatment first hand. We encountered many of the side effects that the majority of patients experience during treatment. We have been presented with different options from our treatment doctors during various phases of our treatment when some of the more not so common side effects reared their ugly heads. Being accustomed to doing research in our own fields, we researched the latest findings from studies conducted relating to those side effects with an emphasis on determining the best routes to take to minimize the impact on our primary treatment, the purpose of which, eradicating the HCV residing in our bodies.

Before beginning treatment, we both found an online support group that consisted of individuals readying for, undergoing, and recovering from HCV treatment. It was our experience that many of these individuals were not very well informed about what to expect, how to react, and options available for issues that arise before, during and after treatment. We want to present to you these most common issues, their cause, their ramifications, and the different options for dealing with those issues, so you can have informed discussions with your doctor with each and every visit as you travel through the treatment process. We will also discuss, in a special section, some rarer, more serious side effects that may be encountered during treatment and the management options of those issues. It is one thing to begin and start the HCV treatment process and quite another to get through it to completion. Our goal is to provide a comprehensive look at the treatment process that will help you conquer the Hepatitis C virus and survive the treatment process.

Chronic HCV now infects 1 in 12 people world wide. HCV infection is the number one cause of cirrhosis, liver failure, liver cancer and liver transplantation. The cost to the health care system is astronomical without factoring in the personal cost to patients when considering loss of work productivity, increased disability, and the impact on the lives of patients and their families. Some reports state there will be an estimated $11 billion spent in direct medical costs. The indirect costs from premature disability and mortality are estimated at $75 billion. These costs will be incurred during the next decade.[1]

The first stage after infection is called acute hepatitis, where there may or may not be symptoms while the body tries to fight off and eradicate the virus with its own immune system. If the body is unable to eradicate (clear) the virus, then the next stage is chronic hepatitis. A full 80% of people go on to experience chronic hepatitis. It is estimated that about 4 million people in the United States are infected with chronic hepatitis C, which is about 2% of the population. This makes HCV much more common than HIV infection.[4] About 2.7 million Americans had chronic Hepatitis C infection in the early 1990s. This number is expected to increase to 10.8 million sometime around the year 2020. Each year, there are about 35,000 cases of acute Hepatitis C and still only 1 in 5, or 20% of those will be expected to clear the virus on their own; the remaining 80% will need to undergo treatment in order to clear the virus and prevent any further possible liver damage caused by the HCV virus.[4]

As we look at treatment and treatment options, we will also examine side effects to treatment and how to counteract those side effects while maintaining a strong offensive toward eradication of the virus. We will also cover the risk each of these issues has on your ultimate chance for successful treatment and achieving a Sustained Viral Response (SVR – undetectable virus 6 months after completion of treatment). It is our primary purpose to educate you to all these issues, so you can be your own best advocate when at a doctor's visit and during your entire course of treatment. This includes treatment modification to deal with side effects as they occur. It is our greatest hope that by making available to you our experiences and research results you will be enabled to speak confidently and in an informed manner to your physician and be a part of the decision making process concerning every aspect of your treatment; in this way you will be capable of maximizing your chances for achieving a sustained viral response.

In this guide, we will take you through the entire process:

- Brief historical perspective of Hepatitis C.
- Getting ready for that first dose of medicine.
- Taking that very first shot.
- The first 4 crucial weeks.
- Through milestone weeks 12, 24, and 48.
- Finally through the post treatment 6-month recovery phase.

Also, included throughout the guide:

- Dealing with and managing adverse side effects.
- Tools to better enable a successful treatment experience.
- Real testimonial stories from patients who have undergone treatment.

We will supply you with tools to make the entire process simpler, help you chart your progress, and continuously track your chances of SVR as you travel through the treatment process. Our hope is for all to achieve SVR status, and while that is an ideal as of this writing, we believe with this helpful guide, you will be enabled to help maximize your chances of conquering Hepatitis C. Our hopes and prayers are with you. Now, prepare to be empowered!

2

History and Epidemiology

Debbie Rae's Story

As cliché as it sounds I believe everything happens for a reason and there are no accidents. One day after years of feeling "toxic" I was determined to put my health at the top of my priority list. Within a few days of my declaration I noticed a red spot on my leg. Then it began to open up to a hole. While driving to report to Jury Duty I was worried about the angry, red hole that was getting bigger on my leg and thought, "wouldn't it be great if I sat next to someone who knew exactly what this was." Well, like I said before, there are no accidents. I was seated next to a friendly man and we got to talking. I showed him my leg and he told me he had been bitten three times by spiders, twice by a Brown Recluse and once by a Black Widow and that my bite was definitely caused by a Brown Recluse.

Not being fond of Western Medicine I have spent my life using alternative therapies and herbal remedies. After his statement I was afraid I would lose my leg since my ex-husband almost lost an arm to a Brown Recluse spider bite, so I immediately sought the help of a doctor. After some blood tests my Dermatologist discovered elevated liver levels and he sent me to an Internist. She informed I tested positive for Hepatitis C. Since I knew nothing of the virus I quickly called a girlfriend and asked, while crying, "should I be scared?" I felt as if someone had just told me I had cancer.

I was on-line that day reading everything I could on Hepatitis C. The one thing I didn't know was how I contracted it. I never used drug needles and didn't have any tattoos but I did have an intensive surgery when I was seven years old and they may have given me a blood transfusion. I also used Cocaine when I was in my twenties and could have contracted it that way. The fact was it didn't matter to me how I contracted it, what mattered was that I had it and my health was in jeopardy. I discovered first hand there was a stigma that came with this virus. I found out it scared people but I didn't care. I was an open book and shared it with all who knew me. Who knows, maybe someday it will come back around and I can help someone else?

By "accident" I was led to one of the best Hepatologists in the U.S. He told me I had "won the lottery" as far as Genotypes; I had Geno 2, a European strain. I believe my lifestyle, regular exercise and a healthy diet, paid off because my viral load was only in the thousands, not millions. My liver was fighting hard to do its job but was continually being attacked by this virus. It was no wonder I felt toxic all the time! My doctor recommended a 6 month protocol of Interferon and Ribavirin. He said my chances of success were 80% versus Genotype 1, which were 50/50. There were new drugs coming down the pike in 2011 but they were targeted for Geno-1. So, I opted for treatment and was anxious to begin.

The side effects were laid out and I was afraid, yet determined. My husband stood solidly by my side. We knew it would be difficult but we knew we could get through it together. I am blessed in that I don't have a job or small children at home to consider, I am retired. In a way, I have the fairy tale story of HCV, if there is such a thing.

Treatment was difficult and I suffered from bouts of migraine headaches, fatigue, fever and chills, skin rashes, mouth sores, changes in appetite, insomnia, shortness of breath, sensitivity to noise, and irritability. The antidepressants that were prescribed a month before treatment helped alleviate the depression but I still had episodes. I believe my bouts of crying were more from exhaustion and feeling poisoned. After about 6 weeks I surrendered to the medication and let it do its "job." The poisonous effects of the drugs took the light out of my spirit and dampened my spark. I felt like a shell, a body with no life force.

The support team I had in place helped carry me through. I joined an on-line forum where other people were going through treatment for HCV. The words I heard throughout were, "it's not forever, just for now." I also had tremendous support from my family and friends. My husband became my biggest hero because he religiously stood by with open arms, no matter how crazy I got. Most importantly he administered my weekly shot and he's scared to death of needles! Sure, we had days that were very difficult. He lost his playmate, his lover, his friend to the drugs and I suffered from exhaustion and felt bad most of the time.

I was what they call an "early responder" and am now "undetectable", just finishing up my treatment. I have three more shots to go out of twenty four. Not only do I believe "there are no accidents" but I also believe "there are gifts or lessons in every adversity." This virus gave me many gifts but the one that stands out as the biggest was learning how to ask for help, knowing my limits and when to say "no", and being able to receive support from loved ones. I took off my superwoman cape and let other people do for me. It was a humbling yet loving act. I hope and pray that anyone who contracts this virus, no matter how they got it, finds the help they need and gets the gift it offers.

With Blessings, Debbie Rae, Cardiff by the Sea, California, April, 2010

Historical Timeline

By 1973, tests had been developed to determine if blood was infected with either the Hepatitis A or Hepatitis B virus. However, there were still cases when patients developed hepatitis after receiving blood transfusions even though the blood they received tested negative for Hepatitis A or Hepatitis B virus. Scientists classified this as yet unknown Hepatitis causing virus as a new mode of developing hepatitis, and gave it a working name of non-A, non-B Hepatitis (NA/NB). Current belief is that perhaps 90-95% of these cases were actually the result of infection by the Hepatitis C virus (HCV).

HCV wasn't discovered until the 1980's; investigators at the Center for Disease Control (CDC), Daniel W. Bradley and Michael Houghton, had finally identified this elusive virus. Blood banks were finally able to start routinely screening blood donors for Hepatitis C in 1990 with a newly developed screening test. Then in 1992, the blood screening test was finally and HCV was effectively cleansed from the nations blood transfusion supply. With the current state of the art testing of the blood supply, today less than one unit in two million are thought to be infected with Hepatitis C virus. It is now believed that prior to this very effective screening process, over 300,000 Americans were infected with the HCV via blood products.

The 1990's saw a period of rapid development and approvals of medications to treat those infected with HCV, beginning with FDA approval of alpha-interferon by Shering. In 1996, Roche received approval of Roferon A to treat HCV. The next year saw FDA approval of consensus interferon (now Infergen by InterMune). The FDA approved Shering's Intron A plus Ribavirin (Rebetron) as a combination treatment therapy for HCV treatment in 1998. Ribavirin is a broad spectrum anti-viral class of drug that was initially developed for the treatment of HIV, but was found ineffective for that purpose. However, Ribavirin was found to be effective in treating HCV, but only in combination with interferon.

The combination of these two drugs was found to provide a synergistic effect, which was deemed a major breakthrough for treating those infected with HCV. The studies conducted with this combination therapy found the best treatment period to be 48 weeks for genotype 1 infected patients and 24 weeks for genotype 2 and 3 infected patients. The response rates for a sustained viral response (SVR) were found to be 29% for genotype 1 and

62% for genotypes 2 and 3. Obviously more effective treatments were needed and continuing research and clinical trials would bring forth even more effective treatment regimens.

The next standard of care developed for treating HCV consisted of a modified form of interferon called pegylated interferon in combination with Ribavirin. Prior to this, patients were required to inject the interferon three times a week. Pegylated interferon stays in the body longer and is injected weekly. This new combination therapy of pegylated interferon and ribavirin improved success rates for SVR. The current SVR rates under this new therapy are approximately 45% SVR for genotype 1 and approximately 80% for genotypes 2 and 3.[1]

Currently in 2010 there have been numerous clinical trials with a new class of drugs that include protease and polymerase inhibitors. They directly interfere with the Hepatitis C virus replication process, and the current results are showing remarkable improvements in SVR rates for genotype 1, approaching those of current rates for genotypes 2 and 3. The first of these drugs, Telaprevir, is anticipated to be available with FDA approval sometime in 2011, if everything goes as currently scheduled.

Epidemiology

The Hepatitis C virus actually comes in different main types, called genotypes. Within the main types there exist sub-types. For example one common main type is genotype "1" and sub-type "a", or more commonly referred to as genotype 1a. Some believe that the HCV virus evolved over thousands of years into these separate genotype versions. This would explain why in different geographical regions different genotypes are more prevalent than in other areas. There are 6 HCV genotypes. In the United States, genotype 1 is the most common accounting for 75% of those infected followed by genotypes 2 and 3 accounting for 22% of infected individuals. Genotypes 3, 4, 5, and 6 are proportionally more prevalent in other parts of the world.[2]

A distinct and major characteristic of Hepatitis C is its tendency to cause chronic liver disease in which the liver injury persists for a prolonged period of time, if not for life. About 80% of patients with acute Hepatitis C ultimately develop chronic infection. Chronic Hepatitis C varies greatly in its course and outcome. At one end of the spectrum are infected persons who have no signs or symptoms of liver disease and have completely normal levels of serum enzymes (the usual blood test results that indicate liver disease). Liver biopsy usually shows some degree of injury to the liver, but the extent is usually mild, and the overall prognosis may be good. At the other end of the spectrum are patients with severe Hepatitis C who have symptoms, high levels of the virus (HCV RNA) in serum, and elevated serum enzymes, and who ultimately develop cirrhosis and end-stage liver disease. In the middle of the spectrum are many patients who have few or no symptoms, mild to moderate elevations in liver enzymes, and an uncertain prognosis.[2]

Modes of Transmission

HCV is spread by blood to blood contact. The historical untested blood supply was a mode of transmission in the past, but with today's screening, this has virtually been eliminated as a mode of transmission. The use of shared, non-sterile needles and other injection paraphernalia is currently the main mode of transmission. However, there are other modes, some being more common than others, one of which is the accidental infection by health care workers during the execution of their job duties. Of the many patients I had the privilege of getting to know undergoing or having completed treatment for HCV, the usual response to origin of contraction was either "I am a healthcare worker (usually a nurse) and have been accidentally stuck over the years on occasion", or "I am a recovering addict, and my past has caught up to me."

Some of the more common risk factors for acquiring Hepatitis C are:

- Injecting drugs, including having used injection drugs only once many years ago.
- Having a blood transfusion before June 1992, when sensitive tests for anti-HCV were introduced for blood screening.
- Receiving clotting factor concentrates (such as anti-hemophilic factor) before 1987, when effective means to inactive HCV were introduced.
- Hemodialysis for kidney failure.
- Birth to an HCV-infected mother (rare).

- Suffering a needle-stick accident from a person infected with Hepatitis C.
- Having sex with someone with Hepatitis C or having multiple sex partners.
- Intranasal use of cocaine using shared equipment or paraphernalia.[2]

Poor medical practices in many parts of the world, such as using medicine vials for delivering multiple doses to more than one individual, reusing syringes, and improperly sterilizing reusable medical equipment leads to medical-care linked transmission of HCV. While these poor practices can be expected from illicit drug users, it should not be tolerated from any medical community, and steps are being taken in an attemp to eliminate this mode of transmission.

Maternal to infant in childbirth does occur, but most studies shows this risk is less than 5%. Sexual transmission also appears possible; surveys indicate that spouses and monogamous relationships where one partner is infected with HCV only have about a 5% incidence rate of both partners being infected. Of course the partners also have other risk factors. Of final note, there is a mode of transmission referred to as *sporadic transmission*. This is the case where no readily common mode of transmission can be identified within an infected individual. This may occur by cuts, accidental exposure during common medical procedures, dental procedures, and the like.[2]

History and Epidemiology

Section References

1. Hepatitis C Support Project.
http://www.hcvadvocate.org/hepatitis/factsheets_pdf/Brief_History_HCV_200
9.pdf

2. http://digestive.niddk.nih.gov/ddiseases/pubs/chronichepc/

3

Diagnosis Process

Lynn's Story

It was the day before Thanksgiving, November, 2005 when I received the call at work that I had Hepatitis C. It was a time of family get-togethers and other than Christmas, one of my favorite holidays of the year. Little did I know that this particular Thanksgiving would change me forever; forever thankful for the many things in life that I had realized, but taken for granted so many years.

I had been experiencing gallbladder attacks for quite some time. Most of the time, the attacks would occur at night after the dinner meal. I had mentioned the pain at my yearly physical and the doctor had informed me when I was ready to be checked for gallstones and have them taken out, to just give him a call. To be honest, I did not really emphasize at the time all the other little symptoms I was having. These symptoms seemed so minor and I thought it was beginning to be part of my life; part of being in a stressful job situation working long hours and hitting those 40's which everyone reminds you changes the way you feel. Most of my day, I would feel pretty good, until late afternoon. By the time I got home in the evening I would be a little shaky feeling-very unlike me. I had always been fairly calm even though my life's events had been everything but calm from the day I sprung into the world. After I would rest an hour or so the jittery feeling would leave me. It would almost be like a feeling you get when you have not eaten all day for some ridiculous reason. I had noticed by Saturday and Sunday I wanted to do fairly little shopping and preferred staying at home and just doing the major chores and resting. That again was atypical of the person I had once been.

Finally, my only daughter and husband convinced me to go back to the doctor since my first grandbaby was due in about two months. I had complained to she and my husband a lot about my minor symptoms but since every morning I "magically" felt better; I had convinced myself life could continue without dreaded surgery.

I contacted my nurse and she referred me to an internist that was close by. I went to her and explained the pain and even admitted to some of the tiredness that I had experienced. She and I agreed that physically I appeared in great shape and probably some of the tiredness was coming from the gallbladder attacks keeping me up at night. She went ahead and did some blood work and said they would contact me soon concerning an ultrasound and probably surgery. I left the office that day not really feeling worried. I always went for yearly check ups and took for granted if there was anything too serious wrong with me that I would have been informed. However, in my heart I knew that there was something wrong with me more than the gallbladder. Your instincts are usually right-you just know when you know. However, I found it easy to try to convince myself otherwise.

About a week later I contacted the doctor's office and spoke with the nurse. She informed me that my liver enzymes were raised about 3 points and they were just asking for additional tests. I asked her what kind of tests and she informed me one was for Hepatitis C. I had been a part time transcriptionist at the hospital for years but knew little about Hepatitis C. My daughter was born in 1978 and I had about 11 blood transfusions at the time due to serious complications from delivery.

My next step I took was to do what everyone else does in this day and age-get on the Internet. After I read the symptoms of Hepatitis C I knew that was what I had. What I did not realize was that you could have it for so many years (27 years in my case) and not know it. A week later I received the call that the test was positive. To say I was upset was an understatement. I left work and went straight to the doctor's office. We conversed for a while and she informed me that they would need to do a viral load test to see if the Hepatitis C was active. I already knew the answer to that question and the viral load came back about 12.5 million. The next step was a liver biopsy and I was informed I was at a Stage II and it was highly recommended that I begin the treatment.

I was so amazed that I had the virus for so many years and it had laid dormant. I never tried any type of drugs and drank on occasion a glass of wine or two with friends or on special occasions. The previous five years had been very stressful; a divorce, hurricane, flood, move, remarriage, job change, family sickness, etc. I guess that includes about all the major stresses one can experience. But, I also realized that it really did not matter how I got the virus-I had it. The major focus for me was to fight with all my life-for my life.

I took the Ribavirin and Interferon shot for 30 weeks. I felt like I had the flu the majority of those weeks; a little achy, low grade fever and tiredness. I worked part of this time and was out on leave part of the time. The hardest thing for me on the first go round of treatment was not feeling like I wanted to eat and being short of breath. The shortness of breath came from my hemoglobin dropping low. The great news was I went into remission in about 12 weeks even with the high viral load. Therefore, after 30 weeks of treatment and losing so much weight they decided to take me off the treatment and see if the virus would stay in remission. In two and a half months the viral load was back up to 2.5 million and a month later it was 5 million. Needless to say, I had to begin the treatment a second go round. Who knows if this would have happened if I could have completed the treatment the first round for the full 48 weeks.

On the third week of treatment on the second round, I lost my father and was absolutely devastated. However, I knew that he wanted nothing in the world more for me than to be well and being the "believer" that I am I was convinced I had another angel on my side. I took Vitamin C and a Multi Vitamin daily, drank about a gallon of water a day, ate fresh fruits and vegetables, prayed and meditated. I put all of my troubles aside and focused entirely on me and the things in life that made me happy. I would imagine on my worst days lying on the beach on a perfect day (not too hot) and watching the waves gently come in and the dolphins dancing in the waters just beyond the shore. I also took the advice of the doctor and took Ambien to sleep at night. I have never been a person that liked to take medicine, but I had been convinced that sleep is extremely important and it is even more so when you body is fighting a virus such as Hepatitis C.

This story has a happy ending. I treated my body with absolute care after coming off the treatment. I realized that was when it was fighting alone without the drugs and I hoped and prayed that the virus would stay permanently in remission. I knew I had age against me, viral load and the amount of time I had the virus. However, I am a 5 foot 1 inch powerhouse when I need to be. When I first found out about the Hepatitis C I read every book I could and gained as much knowledge as possible to fight this monster. I once read a statement where a lady said that it was the worse and best thing that ever happened to her. Now, two years in remission, I understand exactly what she meant. I have changed my life in many ways. I no longer work at the stressful job and every day is a gift. I always had my priorities straight in my head but now I am living those priorities, one by one, day by day. To have Hepatitis C and to fight it is to be true to yourself and to learn who you are and where you want to be *in life. I not only conquered this terrible disease but I conquered myself in the meantime; making each day count and finally living the life I was truly meant to live. Though I started out this journey questioning how could this happen to me at Thanksgiving; I now realize that everyday is Thanksgiving for all of us that are alive, and I know I am truly blessed.*

Lynn

Typical Ways of Discovering Infection

The usual way people discover they have Hepatitis C is through blood testing. How an individual comes to get that testing varies from person to person. Many times there are no symptoms leading one's doctor to do the test that would determine the presence of HCV antibodies. The following is a list of typical situations leading to the discovery of HCV infection.

You're not feeling well, so you see your health care provider who orders blood tests and they find abnormal results. Those abnormal results are usually elevated liver enzymes.

You're feeling well, see your health care provider who orders routine blood tests and you have abnormal results, again usually elevated liver enzymes.

You go to the local blood drive to give blood, and you get a letter saying your blood isn't acceptable for use because they've found HCV antibodies and you need to see your health care provider for follow up.

While applying for life insurance you have a routine checkup, including blood tests, and you are turned down because HCV antibodies are found.

You have read about the risk factors for contracting HCV and decide you want to get yourself tested, and the results come back positive for HCV antibodies.

What Happens Next

When your blood tests come back positive for Hepatitis C antibodies, the next step is to follow up with your primary care provider (PCP). It is critical to be completely honest when answering questions; this aides in diagnosis and prognosis and guides further testing. Getting an idea of when exposure might have occurred indicates length of time of the virus and helps to gauge the degree of possible liver disease. Of course, one must also take into consideration the person's current state of health.

Usually, the next step is to have a baseline viral count done. This is critical because approximately 20% of people clear the virus themselves, without treatment, however they will still test positive for the anti-bodies. This is very important, because if there is no identifiable viral load, then no treatment is necessary. If virus is present, more testing will be done to identify the viral genotype because this has a direct impact on treatment options. You will also find that they will do other blood work as well, to check on your overall well-being and health status.

Depending on the results, you'll want to find out how comfortable your health care provider is in dealing with treatment of HCV. Never feel bad about asking for a consultation with a specialist. Usually, HCV treatment is administered by healthcare professionals who specialize in HCV treatment. Having the blood tests data to give to the specialist is very efficient. Getting a liver biopsy or ultrasound while waiting for the referral to a specialist will give the specialist or your own PCP more data to make informed choices. Facts decrease guesswork. The grade and stage of your liver can have an impact on the likelihood of a successful treatment outcome.

To Treat or Not to Treat

Having confirmed you have chronic HCV infection, and have all your blood test and diagnostic results from such procedures as an ultrasound or liver biopsy, you will meet with your doctor. You and your doctor will discuss whether or not treatment is indicated for your particular case. Some questions you may want to ask in helping you fully understand your situation are listed here:

- Do I have acute or chronic Hepatitis C?
- What are my chances of clearing the virus if I receive treatment?
- What is the chance of me developing cirrhosis or liver cancer if I do not receive treatment?
- What treatment do you recommend? What do I need to know about my treatment?
- How long will I need to be treated? When can I expect to see the results from the treatment?
- How will you assess whether the treatment is working for me?

- What should I do if I have side effects? Is there anything I can take to help the side effects go away?
- Do I have to stop drinking alcohol even if I only have a few beers or a glass of wine once a week?
- How will my Hepatitis C affect my family and friends?
- We want to have kids, is it safe to get pregnant?
- Should I take any special precautions to avoid infecting others?[1]

Section References

1. American Liver Foundation. http://www.liverfoundation.org/education/info/hepatitisc/

4

Readying for Treatment

Spider's Story

I went to the Dentist in January 2008, to have an abscessed tooth pulled, but he would not pull it because my Blood Pressure was too high, so he sent me to my regular Doctor. She did some Blood Tests and discovered elevated liver enzymes! So, she did a complete blood work up and discovered Hepatitis-C Liver Disease, and then my doctor discussed with me a liver biopsy! I'll say at this point I was apprehensive and afraid of the biopsy as well! Being Unemployed and no insurance did not help either. And I'll admit I was in total denial (did not want to believe it)! Why me? - You know the deal.

So, we did the biopsy February 2008 which confirmed it! My Doctor referred me to a local clinic that had a Nurse Practitioner who ran the Hepatitis-C Clinic here in Connecticut. We determined I had got it from a transfusion I had received due to a bleeding ulcer I had back in 1984! I never did the needles or got the Tattoos or had a partner that had it to my knowledge. I did check. I asked my nurse why the Red Cross never picked it up and she said back then there was no test for Hepatitis-C! And there are no symptoms either! We agreed I would start my treatment on April 11, 2008.

My beginning Viral Load was (1,670,000), (SGPT=ALT was 39)! The results of my liver biopsy were moderate degree of Chronic Portal Hepatitis-C - (Genotype 1b). As, I said at first I was in denial and could not find any support groups nearby, so I typed "Hepatitis C" in Google and found the O.A.S.I.S clinic in California online and then found the HCVadvocate.org website where I read Martha's Story and E-mailed her and she became my personal advocate who answered all my questions!

My nurse recommended 48-weeks of treatment with Peg-Interferon and Ribavirin. On Friday April 11, 2008, I took my first shot and Ribavirin and they hit me like a brick wall! I developed a headache, fever, chills, muscle aches and pains, joint pain, and stomach pain! Second week I became anemic and very sensitive to my meds. I became nauseous, throwing up and had trouble breathing (Oxygen- Low) walking up hills. Nurse had to lower Ribavirin dose from 1200 mgs per day down to 800 mgs per day and also ordered Neupogen-1 and Procrit because my hemoglobin took a dive.

This was a life changing event for me! I was losing my hair, my appetite, and weight! Could not have worked even if I had wanted to! I could not sleep in a regular bed and had to sleep in my recliner sitting up! Just the smell of food made my stomach upset. I also had bouts of Depression! (Riba)!

I finished treatment on March 06, 2009 I developed side effects (Post Treatment) that lasted until Sept 2009, which were muscle aches and pains in joints. My viral load check on August 28th, 2009 resulted in "SVR" (50) or below!! My viral load was checked again in December

2010 - results were Non Detectable!! So far I have beat the Dragon with a little Help from my online Hepper Friends! Yayyyyyy!! Every person who decides to treat Hepatitis C is different and reacts differently and I am not a Doctor! If you asked me if it was all worth it, I would say, "HECK YEAH and would treat again if I had to! "

Keep on Keeping On!
Spider123

Believe it or not, there are some things you can do to improve your chances of achieving a sustained viral response (successful treatment outcome), even before you begin treatment. In this section we will look at pre-treatment predictors of a successful treatment response, sometimes referred to as response indicators. We will also look at other things to do to get you ready to embark upon your battle with the HCV that has invaded your body. It will be much better to perform these tasks prior to beginning treatment, when you have the most energy to carry them out. While some people have few or little side effects from treatment, most do experience some or all of the common side effects at one time or another during their course of treatment. We will describe what those are and the availability of over the counter (OTC) medications to help provide symptomatic relief. You will also want to take care of some housekeeping issues and get organized to help you follow your progress through your treatment process. By considering and performing the following suggestions, you will be readying yourself to be fully prepared once treatment begins.

Common Side Effects

As Spider mentioned in his story, he was like many who experience some of the many common side effects to HCV treatment medications. I would like to emphasize here that anyone can suffer through a headache for a day without resorting to taking an over the counter pain reliever, such as acetaminophen, or aspirin. However, treatment lasts a very long time, and to get through it, one must absolutely have a plan for side effect management and the capability to carry that plan out. Don't be a martyr here; you will experience side effects, so be prepared to deal with them and then don't ignore them, but implement your strategies when they occur. To prepare for these side effects it will be helpful to understand how to perform proactive preventative measures to minimize their impact and to learn what over the counter (OTC) remedies are available to help minimize their severity. Here is a list of some of the more common side effects and thoughts on dealing with them.

Fatigue or Tiredness – Treatment is very demanding on the body. Get as much rest as possible whenever the opportunity presents itself. Any amount of exercise you can perform will also help combat fatigue. Insomnia is experienced by some, if not many of those on treatment. Talk to your doctor ahead of time to be prepared in case insomnia becomes an issue for you. Many times your doctor can prescribe something that will help with insomnia or suggest good over the counter alternatives.

Anxiety or Depression – Depression during treatment is a serious issue. A certain percentage of those on treatment will experience clinical depression. Some will at some point feel overwhelmed at the longevity of treatment, and feel blue. Discuss this with your doctor prior to beginning treatment. Some doctors actually prescribe mild anti-depressants as a prophylactic measure. I was prescribed a mild anti-depressant, Trazadone, for a period of time during treatment. I was having insomnia and bouts of mood swings, where I would almost cry at the simplest of things. The Trazadone helped me be able to sleep and moderated my emotions.

Appetite Loss – Many experience side effects that cause foods to taste "strange." There were times when anything I ate tasted very metallic; other times, food tasted just fine, and there was no predicting when these effects would come about. So, when you have an appetite, eat as healthfully as you can. Take vitamins according to your doctor as well. When you do not have an appetite at all, eat smaller healthy meals more frequently during the day.

Indigestion – Try to avoid spicy and other foods that do not agree with your stomach. Ginger ale, and water, and other healthy fluids that are gentle on the stomach should be the mantra. Some have commented that green tea appeared to help them with many of the side effects of treatment.

Insomnia – As mentioned before, trouble sleeping often comes at times during treatment. Getting enough rest is crucial to feeling as good as possible and having the energy to do the things we absolutely need to get done.

Discuss using over the counter sleep aids or prescribed medications with your doctor to help ensure you get the rest you need.

Cognitive Thinking Loss – This is commonly referred to as "brain fog." It is a feeling of being unable to think very clearly; inability to concentrate, and forgetfulness are others symptoms commonly associated with "brain fog." Not getting enough water can exacerbate this problem. It is very important to get enough clear fluids during treatment. For those who have not built up a tolerance to caffeine, caffeinated beverages can act as a diuretic causing fluid loss. It is best to drink only clear fluids, such as water and sugarless sports drinks. Electrolyte replacement is also very important during treatment, so talk to your doctor about the best ways to ensure you maintain a healthy electrolyte balance in your system.

Other Side Effects – The side effects of treatment are many and varied. I am sure there are more not listed here. Always consult your doctor about side effects you experience. Keep a journal as you experience them and then if serious call your doctor right away. Take your journal with you to each doctor's visit. This will also allow you to have a notebook available to take notes during your visits.

Online Support Group

If knowledge is power, then to know a thing is to have power over it. Before leaping into a fray, it would best serve one to turn on a light by which to see. By looking around and studying the surroundings, it will greatly help in the acquisition of one's goal. Similarly, to tread alone a weary and obstacle ridden path, will surely lead to exhaustion and possible folly; whereas to grab hold of one who also seeks your destination to steady each other along the way will create power in a synergistic fashion to enable both to overcome even the most dangerous of pitfalls. To this end, we, the authors, embarked upon a journey to better enable the fruition of these ideals when it comes to HCV treatment. The idea is that this book will be the immediate source of knowledge compiled in a nice organized concise manner. The online support forum that is the co-companion to this book will provide the means for those undergoing treatment to journey together, helping each other along the way, providing and receiving support that is so very helpful. We hope you will join the forum and follow in the footsteps of our fearless founders who have so clearly marked a wonderful path to take. If you want to participate in the ongoing support that helps so much in undergoing HCV treatment, please visit and join the membership free support forum at www.hcvshare.org.

Pre-treatment Indicators of Success

BMI and Steatosis

There's not much one can do about their race or age or some of the other pre-treatment indicators, however, there is something one can do about their weight prior to and during treatment. Obesity is defined by a certain level of the Body Mass Index (BMI). It is dependent upon ones waist measurement, and the measurement of actual body fat content. Studies indicate that obese patients do not respond as well as those individuals with a healthy BMI. So, the closer one is to an ideal body weight, the more one improves their chances for a successful treatment outcome or sustained virological response. An associated condition to body fat is steatosis. Steatosis is the result of fatty infiltrates building up in the liver, which can not only speed up disease progression, but have a negative impact on treatment response. To combat steatosis, one should maintain a healthy lifestyle, eating a healthy diet, and exercising regularly. In patients without steatosis the SVR rate was 61.2% but in patients with steatosis SVR was achieved in 102 of 215 (46.6%) patients; P<0.001.[1] that is a relative improvement from 46.6% of 31%!

Alcohol

While on treatment it is recommended that everyone abstain from drinking alcohol. Pegylated Interferon and Ribavirin therapy for HCV has been associated with relapse for those patients who have a history of drug or alcohol abuse. The typical recommendation is for a prospective patient who has a history of alcohol abuse to have not used alcohol six months prior to beginning treatment. Practicing alcohol or drug abusers can be successfully treated, but treatment should be in conjunction with ongoing counseling with alcohol or drug abuse specialists or counselors. Even prospective patients on a methadone program can be successfully treated, although close coordination needs to be administered in case there is a need to modify the methadone prescription while on HCV treatment.[2]

Drinking alcohol is or should be considered one of the worst things you could do prior to and during treatment. It is well known that continual drinking of alcohol leads to liver damage, and exacerbates the effects that HCV has on the liver. In regards to the effect on treatment, the anti-HCV action of interferon-alfa was reduced in the presence of ethanol (Alcohol), most likely via attenuation of Stat1 tyrosine-701 phosphorylation. Even more importantly, it has been found that those on treatment who drank alcohol within the past year prior to starting treatment had a much higher rate of treatment discontinuation than those who did not drink alcohol (40% vs. 26%; P = 0.0002) and a trend toward a lower SVR rate (14% vs. 20%; P = 0.06). [3]

Vitamins

A remarkable study recently showed very good promise on the synergistic effects of Vitamin D along with Pegylated Interferon and Ribavirin treatment in increasing the Rapid Viral Response of patients undergoing therapy for HCV. A Rapid Viral Response is defined as having undetectable HCV in blood serum at the 4 week mark after beginning therapy. At the 2009 Annual Meeting of the American Association for the Study of Liver Diseases (AASLD), Saif M. Abu-Mouch, M.D., from the Department of Hepatology, Hillel Yaffe Medical Center in Hadera, Israel reported, "This preliminary study confirms the benefit of adding Vitamin D to conventional antiviral therapy in patients with chronic Hepatitis C." A control group was given standard of care treatment and a separate group was also given Vitamin D 1000 to 4000 IU daily. The control group had an 18% RVR rate, while the vitamin D group had a 44% RVR response rate. At week

12, 96% of the vitamin D group had achieve undetectable HCV, while only 48% of the control group were undetectable. These results are very remarkable and point to an also remarkable increase in ultimate SVR (or cure) rate for those individuals who insure proper Vitamin D levels in their system. It should be noted that Vitamin D is fat soluble and taking too much Vitamin D can lead to serious issues, so as always, consult with your doctor before treatment and get permission to take Vitamin D at the maximum allowed dose your doctor will allow and prescribe.[4]

Other Ways to Prepare

One of the very first things you will want to do is a very good spring cleaning of your house. During treatment, many times you will not have the energy or motivation to perhaps do a thorough and proper job of your everyday chores. Also, outside work chores that may have been put off until now should be done. While many still do perform routine chores such as lawn maintenance and such while on treatment, there will most likely be little motivation to perform those extra items such as that needed fence mending, or roof repair. Take care of all those issues prior to starting treatment, so you don't have to worry about that leaky drip in the roof when the winter rains come around. Minimizing these possible stressors as much as possible will allow you to focus on your treatment and focus on what is really important; looking after your treatment and making sure you stay in adherence as much as absolutely possible is your #1 priority.

This would also be a great time to discuss with any one who you feel should know about your upcoming treatment, explain to them the side effects you will be experiencing, and rally as much support as you can from those close to you that will be able to help out in even the slightest way, when your needs call upon them. There may be times, when you might need a ride to a doctor's visit or need someone to pick up something for you, when you just do not feel that you can get out of the house.

It will be very helpful throughout treatment to have and keep a journal of your treatment. Not only is "brain fog" (periods of lack of concentration or impaired cognitive ability) a very real side effect during treatment, but the extended length of treatment alone calls for keeping good records during the process. Here you can also keep a list of questions to ask your physician and write down the answers, so you can refer back at the appropriate time. During treatment, you will experience a side effect, and when that happens, write down the specifics, including your feelings and perceptions, as well as what you were doing just prior, and any other details; then when you next talk to your physician, you will be well prepared.

Be sure to set aside a separate folder (or folders) for keeping your paperwork organized, in duplicate if possible; for instance, you will want a folder for insurance records, medication receipts, lab results, and any other specific or general reports. By keeping track of these items, you will be able to compare one lab results to a previous one, to see how you are trending; whether you are maintaining a steady level, improving, or perhaps going in a direction that should be watched closely.

Blood lab tests are performed quite often during treatment. Generally your viral load count and thyroid stimulating hormone (TSH) will be tested just prior to treatment and at weeks 4, 12, 24, 48, and 24 weeks post treatment. After the first 4 weeks of treatment, about every 4 weeks thereafter, your complete blood count (CBC with differential), liver enzymes (ALT/AST), and HCG (if fertile) will be monitored as well.

Section References

1. http://www.natap.org/2008/HCV/031008_01.htm

2. http://digestive.niddk.nih.gov/ddiseases/pubs/chronichepc/index.htm

3. McCartney, Erin, et. Al., *Journal of Infectious Diseases*, Dec 15, 2008 (http://www.janis7hepc.com/effects_of_alcohol_hcv_treatment.htm)

4. http://www.hepatitis-central.com/mt/archives/2009/12/could_vitamin_d.html

5

That Very First Shot

Mynnie's Story

January 20, 2010

In 2001, I was living on a boat in Marina Del Rey, had a great job in West Hollywood, ran on the beach every day, and finally had health insurance. This was a good time to go for a full physical, including blood tests. I called back as requested to follow up on the lab results, and they wanted me to come back in, to do more blood work. Why? "To rule out Hep C." What? Rule it OUT? Well, I certainly did not want to take the chance of ruling it IN! This might mean I'd have to stop my "secret life" of drinking and using. So I did not go back.

For the next couple years, my life went downhill. I was pretty much forced, by dire circumstances, to pull my life together and get clean and sober. By this time, I'd ended up in a tiny little town in the mountains in northern California. Eventually, I again found myself with a job and insurance, so decided it was time to face the facts. I went to a doctor, told him I may have Hep C., and did the blood work again. Yes. I decided to take the bull by the horns and get treatment. This was in 2004. I was sent to a specialist, had a biopsy (completely uneventful) and was told that I was a good candidate for treatment. My biopsy showed the beginnings of cirrhosis. That is all I really knew besides the fact that I did have Hep C. There was no mention of genotypes, or viral loads. I had no idea what to expect, beyond the fact that I might not feel well for a while. I'd never known anyone who'd had the disease or gone through treatment.

My first shot seemed to go OK initially. I had decided that I would continue my life just the same as before the shot, no matter what. Immediately I was consumed with a total lack of energy, along with depression so severe that I went from being a naturally happy person, to one who was choked up and likely to cry at any given moment. Still, I continued to run my dog 3 or 4 miles a day, and kept up all other social and work obligations, determined to persevere. The day after my second shot, I left on a business trip to Chicago, and it was there, after a few days of things going wrong, that I looked out my 17th floor hotel window and suddenly jumping out sounded like a good idea. That is how down I was.

I took a couple steps back in my mind. "WHAT the @#%!" I've never been suicidal in my life, no matter HOW DOWN. I stopped the Riba pills that night, and decided that even if I had 10 years left on my life, I was going to live them med free. I did not want to waste one more minute feeling miserable on this poison. When I told my doctor, after returning home, that I was not going to continue treatment, he suggested going to a half dose of everything, but my mind was made up.*

Four years passed, with me living a pretty good life, in a great, all-eclipsing state of denial. I worked, I traveled abroad many times, skied, ran, mountain biked, swam, and generally enjoyed my life. A friend was an Aruveydec Practitioner, and I went on the herbal remedy she prescribed. I also worked with a life coach who told me that I could get rid of Hep C by visualizing myself virus free. My wake up call came in the fall of 2008. After participating in a mini-triathlon, there was no runner's high and instead it seemed to take a few months to recover. I was exhausted all the time, and a feeling of lethargy replaced my usual energy. I knew it was the Hep C. A few months before, I joined the HCV Support website and had begun educating myself and reading the posts that others sent in sharing their experience. I realized that I needed to seek treatment, and once on it, I had to commit to it.

By now, I was an independent contractor, living job-to-job, with no insurance, and no more money in the bank. I wrote about my situation on the site, and began getting suggestions. A clinical trial seemed like it would be the best avenue. Upon screening for the two clinical trials that I applied for, I learned that, though in every other way I was a good candidate, I happened to have Genotype 3 and so could not participate. Most studies are for 1, as it is the most challenging to cure. I was devastated. I also learned my viral load at that time: 7 million.

By this time, my Mom knew, too. We were both so upset, as the clinical trials had looked so promising. The good news was that I would require only 6 months treatment rather than the usual year and that my success rate was higher. I'd been to South America many times and had friends there who looked into all costs for getting treatment down there. My mother said she would loan me up to a certain amount of money. The response was disappointing: even down there, treatment and living costs would come to much more than we could afford.

I posted all of this on the HCV site. So far, it seemed like one avenue after the other had closed. My application for government medical assistance was denied because I was working and making too much to qualify. $18,000 a year, evidently, put me over the top. It was suggested that I try the patient assistance programs at the pharmaceutical companies. I started with a phone interview. They sent forms to be completed by my doctor, and I had to verify the last year's income. Within about 3 weeks of my initial contact, I received 4 pre-filled Pegasys shots and a month's worth of the Copegus pills by Fed Ex.

I now knew that there were ways to counteract almost all of the sides. Due to the depression I had experienced before, my doctor put me on an anti-depressant for one month prior to starting treatment.

At first, because I was working, I was coming out of pocket, though it was tough, for lab tests including weekly blood tests. (We found out the first time around that I was prone to having my white blood cell count drop, so the doctor was keeping a close eye on me.) The third week, after getting my blood drawn, I commented to the receptionist that it was hard for patients like me, kind of falling into the cracks of our current medical system. If you have a "Pre-existing condition" for one, the cost of medical insurance shoots up so high as to make it impossible to afford. If you have no insurance, but you are working and make a little money, you can't qualify for aid. And the $268 I was paying almost weekly was really hard to scrape up. The woman I said that to, right then and *there made a phone call to the head of the hospital's billing department, and a meeting was set up for me to go talk to them that day. The outcome was that I did not have to pay for any more labs thanks to a charitable foundation set up for people just like me. I almost cried! Also, when I let my doctor's office know that I was paying cash, my visits went from $80 to $50. For any other prescriptions I needed, I phoned around and found a discount pharmacy and always got the generic version, when available.*

Many people work through treatment, and I am one of them. I promote and run trade shows all over the country, and also plan local events. Even when not on meds and feeling great, this is a grueling job. For me, there was no choice BUT to work, as I am an independent contractor, with no other income. I also cannot afford to lose my reputation for being good at my job, as I have a lot of competitors bidding on the work I get.

Working and traveling through treatment was unspeakably hard. As luck would have it, I suddenly landed every job I'd bid on earlier in the year. In the 24 week period that I was on treatment, I promoted and ran 14 shows, many times flying or driving from one city to the next, in addition to 2 local weddings.

I had to find it in myself to put on a spunky persona, which somewhat resembled my former self, when running a show and interacting with vendors, or when going into the office to drop off materials and reports. I'd have to try not to itch (riba rash – bad for 2 months), cover up any skin that showed (bumps all over),and fluff off the fact that I'd cut off my long blond hair in favor of a sassy short cut (that better covered the bald spots on my head).

Somehow I never missed a plane, and never had a bad show. I'd get home for a day or a week and collapse.

A few times I suffered total meltdowns. One time stands out. I worked all week promoting a show in Columbus, Ohio, then was on-site coordinator for show day, and that night drove 3 hours, stuck in traffic to Cincinnati, so I could run a show there the next day. When I arrived at my hotel in Cincinnati, I was exhausted, my throat hurt, every part of me ached, and I had a fever. I felt I could not go on, but after an all-out sobbing episode, and a talk with one of my friends at home, I calmed down enough to get some rest before my 5am wake-up.

For my last few months on treatment, I had a friend from HCV support who accompanied me "virtually" on my trips. Every time I got home to my computer, I'd touch base with my buddies on the HCV site. The understanding, support and encouragement I got from these fellow "heppers" got me through.

I kept a journal throughout the whole experience. During treatment, I was reluctant to share my worst moments with others, as I did not want to deter someone from seeking treatment. Now that I am done, I will share just one line from an entry, Week 15 of Treatment, Day 2 (I was in the middle of a 2 week, 2 city work trip):

"I have fear this headache is dimming all light in my day, that my life is only drudgery, and no light at all."

The next week I got the results of my viral load test – I was undetectable, which helped me to keep plugging along. My blood cell counts, both red and white, were dropping. Near the end they declined into what the doctor considered "dangerous levels." Week 22, I was just returning from my last shows of the year, and my lab results were not good. I'd been on reduced meds since week 16, and by week 23, the doc said there were no other options: I had to stop treatment. By this time, my head was killing me, and I could barely peel myself out of bed to go get a blood test.

My viral load post treatment was undetectable; Whew. By this time, I felt as though a tornado had picked me up, thrashed me around for 6 months, and then dropped me down. The new me was a wreck, emotionally, physically and mentally. For the first week, I felt that, yes, it was wonderful that I was well, but then I went through a spell of feeling acutely aware of and embarrassed by my short thinning hair, unsightly rash everywhere, loss of muscle tone, puffiness, bloating, and dark circles under my eyes. You don't care about stuff like that when you are on the treatment and just lucky to be out doing your job. I had to work on a better attitude about it all, but the work paid off.

I am now almost 7 weeks post treatment; the "old" me is coming back. I have learned so much through this experience, and the lessons I've learned I would not trade for anything. I've learned that I am not defined by how I look on the exterior. I am so much more than that. I feel as if a huge chunk of self-focus was carved out of me, making room for large amount of giving to others. It deepened my capacity for compassion, and patience, with others and me. I learned to really, and I mean REALLY pay attention to my body and state of mind, and to take care of both. I learned that I am strong and courageous, and, with the help of others, can make it through almost anything. And good health, good frame of mine, and life itself, are not to be taken for granted. Being alive is GLORIOUS!

Mynnie

Anxiety and Expectations

Most individuals who have been given the go ahead by their treating physician to begin treatment, immediately start to get a little anxious about starting treatment. They worry how the medications will affect them specifically; will they experience few side effects, or will they be one who experience many side effects? Will they be able to continue to work and function, both inside the home, and out? Will they become an extra burden on their loved ones? For those living alone with little support, will they be OK at home alone taking these medications? Mynnie's story really gives us insight into these thoughts, and shows us how one person dealt with these issues.

The anxiety and fear that come with the unknown are natural reactions and these are all very valid questions to ask. It might help to know that many individuals do continue to work while on treatment, and find that they are fully capable of continuing to perform chores around the house. Some, however, do end up taking time off from work or even family medical leave or going on temporary disability for certain periods during treatment. One thing for certain is that worrying unnecessarily will not change what is to come.

However, by preparing ahead of time for such events, should they occur, will enable one to feel confident and prepared, thus removing any anxiety that might be present due to being unprepared. So, check into your work's family leave policy. Talk with your spouse about a plan if your side effects become more debilitating than most experience. Connect with your support system to make sure someone will be available to help you if the need arises.

Administering Medications

There is a traditional syringe and vial approach delivery system for the Pegasys portion of the treatment regimen and also the Pegintron Powder for the Redipen, which is an easy to use pen delivery system. Your treating physician should decide which system is best for your particular situation. There are also two types of Pegylated Interferon currently being used for treatment regimens, however, a study reported in the New England Journal of Medicine showed there was no appreciable difference in SVR rates for the different regimens.[1]

It is very important to remember to have food on your stomach when you take your Ribavirin medication. It can be helpful to take your dose after the morning meal and after the evening meal to get into a regular routine. As for the first shot of the Pegylated Interferon, many have found that the side effects do not occur until hours after taking the shot; so some will take the shot in the morning to be able to meet any side effects while still awake; others choose to take the shot in the evening, take acetaminophen if approved by their doctor, and then sleep any side effects away. I personally had body aches and mild fever (just like the flu) about 10 hours after taking my first shot. I took 2000mg acetaminophen (approved by my doctor), and felt fine soon after; I never had any side effects like these on subsequent shots. Many indicate the immediate side effects from the first shot are usually worse than subsequent shots.

You may be required to take a class on how to administer the medications. Ribavirin is taken orally, but the Pegylated Interferon is administered subcutaneous (under the skin in the fatty section). You will be trained on how to administer your shot of Pegylated Interferon, and after the first couple, should become very adept at self-administering. The Pegasys medication guide includes a location chart indicating injection locations on the abdomen and upper thighs; please refer to that guide and your doctor for a complete description of location sites and methods of administration.[2]

Organization of Medications

One of the causes of relapse and non-response to treatment is due to non-compliance to treatment protocol. Ribavirin dosage is based on the weight of the individual. Ribavirin is usually taken twice a day, while the Pegylated Interferon is taken as a weekly injection. The treatment protocol is defined as the prescribed dosages of medications and frequencies of administration. If a person forgets to take one of the daily doses of Ribavirin, this can lead to a diminished concentration of medicine within one's body. While one missed dose may not affect a statistical outcome in overall treatment response, this can become a bad habit or a frequent occurrence, and that could very well lead to a difference in outcome.

To offset this danger of becoming non-compliant to protocol, there are a few things one can do to help decrease the risk. One very simple tool is to use an AM/PM Weekly pill container. Each week, if you fill this container with the following week's medications and other doctor approved supplements, such as Vitamin D, it will be simple to determine if you have taken your morning or evening dose for that day. The first time I had to empty my Ribavirin bottle and count up all the remaining pills to see if I had taken my current dose, I purchased one of these wonderful simple inexpensive tools. There are also, medication alarm watches that you can set for multiple times a day as a reminder to take your medication.

While you can keep your Ribavirin in an organized pill container, you will need to keep your Pegylated Interferon refrigerated. The insert for the medication of Pegasys calls for keeping the medication within a certain temperature range, and to ensure that the medication is not frozen. Please refer to the medication insert for the exact temperature range. There is a number to call, listed in the insert, should you question whether your medication has been compromised by inadequate storage methods. Even though, you are unlikely to forget whether you have taken the current week's shot of Pegylated Interferon, you should still keep a journal record of your shots, including the date and time of injection.

Section References

1. N Engl J Med. 2009 Aug 6;361(6):580-93. Epub 2009 Jul 22
http://www.ncbi.nlm.nih.gov/pubmed/19625712?dopt=abstract

2.
http://www.gene.com/gene/products/information/pegasys/pdf/Pegasys_MedGuide.pdf

6

Weeks 1-4

Hop's Story - How to be a hero

"We can be hero's... just for one day." - David Bowie

There was little in my life that could have prepared me for the phone call from my primary care doctor of 25 years. In a calm, matter of fact voice he told me that my liver enzymes were highly elevated, meaning that there was a problem we had to investigate further. He wanted me to have more blood drawn for another battery of tests. When I said I was swamped with work and would get to it next week, he said, "No. Do it tomorrow." He was candid about many of the possible sources of the elevation, none good.

I'm not giving away the ending when the next call told me I was Hepatitis C positive, which now required additional blood work to double check the results, determine genotype and gauge viral load. I had no clue about the nature of the disease. I was scared.

I had experienced a myriad of strange symptoms for so many years, that they had become part of who I was. Migraines, insomnia, 'car sickness', contact dermatitis, blurred vision dizziness and night sweats among others, well before menopause would be a factor. It was when I developed a vertigo that didn't resolve, that they finally dug deeper and discovered the HCV. The doctors said that most of these pesky complaints were probably underlying HCV symptoms all along, although they couldn't say for sure.

A common experience for many of us has been, "What just happened? I went to my doctor's office relatively healthy and left with a diagnosis of HCV that will change my life. How did this happen?" As a healthy, non-risk taking, non-smoking, non-drinking, non-substance, health-conscious female, I always felt impervious. Not that my life has been charmed or easy, not by a long shot. But my world had evolved into a happy, contented, privileged place of family, close friends, lots of travel and work I loved.

Having most likely acquired the HCV, genotype 1b, during a series of surgical procedures for endometriosis between 26-30 years ago, not knowing the 'how or when' of my exposure drove me so batty for those first few weeks, that I couldn't think about much else - other than finding out as much as I could about the disease itself.

When I finally realized that how I got it was placing emphasis on something I couldn't change, I focused instead on finding the right doctor and my exploring treatment options. Almost immediately, I knew I would opt for treatment, as I would never be any younger or healthier than I was at that moment.

The virus changed my world. Even before I began to treat, I had to become someone else; Someone who had to fight for ever crumb. Someone who needed to read about and research every imaginable disease permutation and *treatment option. A reluctant, yet heroic fighter who had to traverse the private insurance systems (both medical and disability) like a pro, fighting every "no" with a "why not?" Fighting to get the right doctor. Fighting for copies of the latest blood results. Fighting for more than seven weeks to get insurance approval for the combination treatment. Fighting to stay optimistic. Fighting for the right to fight.*

I began the standard of care, combination treatment of Pegylated Interferon/Ribavirin approximately six months after my diagnosis. Like many, my narrow world now revolves around the treatments. How do I feel today? How will I feel this evening? Can I sleep? Am I drinking enough? Why does everything taste like metal? When will the doctor call? Is that more hair falling out? Can I make it up the stairs? Can I work? What do I say to family who want to know how I'm doing today? What has happened to my social life? All I want to do is crawl under a rock. Who knew that this fight could be so demanding?
My world has reduced down to very bare essentials.

Now in treatment, I've become exhausted from anemia, shortness of breath, insomnia and muscle aches, along with some of the more exotic side effects. Reluctantly, I've come to the realization that I won't be able to muscle through this on sheer will power and resilience for 48 weeks after all. I have to keep fighting. I've had to learn to be a hero.

For reason that I now recognize as sheer hubris, I thought that I would be impervious to the side effects that others suffered from during treatment. I sailed right through the first three weeks, but now appreciate that all of the changes, day-to-day and hour-to-hour, are the new normal.

I am not currently able to work, which affects my self-image. Although optimistic and sunny by nature, I have too much time to mourn the person I used to be, while simultaneously discovering the person I am fighting to become. Friend's call, needing me to reassure them that everything is normal. All I can think about is my shortness of breath and how long I can talk without getting too tired, challenging my perceptions of who I am in the world.

In my typically optimistic fashion, though, I keep waiting for some really cool Super Hero version of the side effects to kick in. After all, isn't this how Super Heroes are born? By foisting some weird toxic chemical cocktail upon a mild-mannered, unsuspecting bystander? I had always pictured that if I were ever to turn into a Super Hero; my side effects would be more along the lines of telekinesis, astral projection or x-ray vision.

If I've learned anything from this ongoing battle, it's that good or bad, each day is a new day, full of new unknowns. I'm also learning how not to be so fearful of the unknown, to build on being as actively accepting as possible; learning how to keep moving forward.

A virus, by virtue of definition, is an infectious agent that replicates. As such, a virus can also infect our minds and our spirits with hopelessness or intolerance; in other words, an insidious predator of mind and body, over which we may have very little control. Similarly, a virus can contaminate our outlook. However painful, how we view our world and how we choose to treat others is something that we can try to manage.

My parents (and most of their friends) are Holocaust survivors who at an early age and through no fault of their own lost everyone and everything to a virus called intolerance. Afterwards, they were compelled to rebuild. I always knew they were heroes; they are certainly mine, but given my experiences grappling with HCV during the past number of months, I now recognize that the most heroic thing that we can do in our lives is continue to fight for those things that make a difference, no matter how tired we become.

This, then, is how we truly become heroes – by getting through each day.
Best to all, both warriors and caretakers, as you learn to fight your personal HCV battles.

Introduction

In this section we are going to discuss the issues that are most relevant to the first four weeks of treatment. It is during this time that you will be thrust from your previous life of living with HCV with as much normality as possible into a life of living with treating the HCV and all that entails. We will first look at what you can do to make this adjustment as painless as possible. Next, we will look at what side effects you are likely to encounter, their possible severity, and solutions to try out to deal with them should the need arise. After that, we are going to look at the topic of "Viral Kinetics." Viral kinetics describes the body's response to treatment in terms of how the virus is eradicated over time from the first week of treatment through the remaining weeks. Finally, we will explore the most frequently looked at results from blood work you will have done during the first four weeks and identify those things that might raise a warning flag and indicate a need to closely follow up on with subsequent blood test results.

Adjusting to Treatment

Most patients are very apprehensive prior to beginning treatment about how their daily activities will change during treatment. One thing for certain is that you will most likely experience many side effects at one time or another during treatment, but in the first few weeks, they will seem more intense than later on. One reason for this is because of the anticipation that has been felt prior to beginning. Another reason is that later on, when you experience side effects, you will most likely have already experienced them and have a plan of attack to deal with them, either in the form of over the counter medications, or from medications prescribed during prior visits to the doctor. Another necessary adjustment will be in household activities such as chores and other daily activities, and employment, if working.

While on treatment, and from the very beginning, many experience mild flu like symptoms, shortness of breath (SOB) and lightheadedness. The mild flu like symptoms can be minimized to a great extent by drinking an appropriate amount of water. It is usually recommended to drink the number of ounces of water equal to half your body weight in pounds daily; for example for a 192lb individual, you should drink about 96 fluid ounces (3 quarts) of water a day. The shortness of breath and light-headedness is usually brought on by the reduced number of red blood cells resulting from Ribavirin-induced anemia. Almost everyone experiences this anemia to one degree or another, however a small percentage of individuals may experience it to a degree that may call on the need for medical intervention in the form of modifying one's treatment; this will be discussed further and in even more depth under the adverse sides effects and management section.

The anemia indicator on the blood test results is referred to as Hgb, which is short for hemoglobin. The level of Hgb is indicative of the degree of anemia if below a certain normal range minimum; a lower number indicates a greater amount of anemia. The shortness of breath (SOB) that one experiences can also be felt as being very easy to tire. However, usually one is also very quick to recover from this feeling, if one sits and rests for a time. Adjustment in the early weeks to this condition will demand finding a balance between performing one's necessary responsibilities and not overextending one's current physical capacity to do work. Once this anemia response sets in, you will quickly find that balance, but it is very beneficial to be aware of it beforehand.

Many individuals who undergo treatment do continue to function and perform their employment obligations both within and outside the workplace. Though often times, it is necessary to adjust at work just as you have learned to adjust at home. Symptoms of anemia can cause problems for those who have physically demanding jobs. It is very difficult to be on one's feet for the majority of the work day while undergoing treatment for those who are experiencing anemia. For those individuals who cannot continue to perform their work functions in an adequate manner, they should consult with their human resources department at work and ask about going on either disability or taking leave, possibly through the Family Medical Leave Act (FMLA).

Early Common Side Effects

Along with the shortness of breath, you will in all probability have to get accustomed to other common side effects. The most likely side effects you may encounter in the first four weeks, aside from shortness of breath, are headaches, mild fever, body aches, diarrhea, dry or sore eyes, mild reaction at the injection site. Dry skin can be caused by the medications and dehydration. You may suffer insomnia, mouth sores or "rawness", angular cheilitis (cracks in corners of mouth), trouble concentrating (brain fog), and possibly a red rash in areas due to the Ribavirin, which many refer to as Riba Rash. As the weeks go by the Riba Rash may worsen. You may experience some hair thinning or loss, and possibly some more serious side effects that will be addressed later..

That may have just sounded like one of those commercials that spout all the possible side effects of a medication to cure a tummy ache. But on HCV treatment, some or most of all the common side effects are experienced by many. For the most part, the less serious symptoms are more of a nuisance than anything else. Most are easily relieved with doctor prescribed or doctor approved medications. We have devoted an entire section to the more serious side effects and their management throughout treatment. As always, be sure to ask your doctor for approval before taking any medications, even over the counter ones.

Viral Kinetics and SVR

Viral Kinetics is the study of how the virus evolves over time. Studies were performed to show how the HCV virus population changes after high dose injections of alfa-interferon. These studies showed two separate phases of virus elimination. The first phase occurs after the first few hours of injection and lasts between 8-12 hours and is attributed to a rapid viral decline, with the second phase lasting days, but with a much slower level of decline.[1] When a patient is undergoing treatment, they are normally taking Pegylated Interferon shots on a weekly basis. This is usually combined with twice daily oral administration of Ribavirin. Combined, these two medications, as of this writing, make up the standard of care treatment. If one were to average the rate of destruction of virus and subtract the average rate of production of new virus, one would know the average rate of decline, and this could be shown as the log drop achieved for a particular week.

For instance, let's suppose that on medication, there are 50% of the virus being destroyed each week and that there are 10% of the virus being replicated each week. We can see that there is a net 40% of the virus being destroyed each week. To calculate the log drop for the week, we would calculate –LOG(100%-40%) = 0.22 LOG Drop. Not everyone will achieve the same rates of destruction or have the same rates of production;

therefore, in treating patients for HCV, a wide variability exists in the observed rates of decline, commonly referred to as log drop, which is nothing more than the Base 10 Log of the ratio of the beginning virus concentration to the ending virus concentration as observed in the blood through a lab test.

So, that was a lot of fairly technical information, so I will try to re-state it more concisely and clearly. During treatment from the beginning to when one finally has no detectable virus in their blood (Undetected), people clear the virus at slower or faster rates, so while some take only a few weeks to be undetected, others take many weeks. If a person does not clear the virus by week 24, they are generally referred to as a non-responder. Also, if a person does not achieve a 99% decline in virus by week 12, they are also generally considered to be non-responsive. One would think that no matter how long it took one to clear the virus, they would still have the same chances of a complete sustained viral response (SVR) as anyone else that cleared and completed a 48 week treatment regimen. However, this is not the case. Indeed it has been shown that the time required to clear the virus is correlated to the chances of SVR as described next.

First we will look at some definitions:

1. RVR – Rapid Viral Response occurs when a person achieves undetectable HCV in the blood by week 4 of treatment (4 weeks after treatment begins).

2. cEVR – Complete Early Viral Response occurs when a person achieves undetected status by week 12.

3. pEVR – Partial Early Viral Response occurs when a person achieves a 10 times decrease (-2 log drop) in HCV blood serum concentration by week 12 and continues to undetectable status by week 24.

The order of response form quicker to slower is RVR, then cEVR, and finally, pEVR. Along this spectrum of responses, their exists different overall responses to treatment with the chances of achieving SVR being greater the more quickly you achieve undetectable status, with the RVR cases having the greatest chance of achieving SVR.[2]

It should be noted here that even though a person may belong to a certain group who has achieved an RVR response and that group has a combined certain statistical likelihood of achieving SVR, does not mean that by looking at any one individual, one would be able to determine beforehand if that person will go on to achieve SVR or not. That is one reason we use statistics in discussing matters such as this. It serves to indicate *on a relative scale* the differences from one group to another. So, when we talk about the chances of SVR here, we are talking about the percentage of a certain group of individuals, not any particular person.

Rapid Viral Responders have a 90% chance of achieving SVR. Early Viral Responders have a 70% chance to go onto and achieve SVR.[2] However early viral responders constitute those who achieve a complete early response (undetectable by week 12) and those who are not undetectable until sometime between weeks 12 and 24; the latter are referred to as partial early viral responders, or sometimes as slow responders. We will look more at these differences in a later section, and also show you how to calculate the statistical likelihood of achieving SVR based on your current particular viral kinetics and statistical probabilities in the tools section.

Week 4 Blood Tests

After week 4 of treatment, there is usually a scheduled doctor visit or blood lab visit to take blood for performing some very important tests to determine how your body is responding to treatment. Ribavirin can cause birth defects, so women who are of reproductive age and fertile must have monthly pregnancy tests and be on two forms of reliable birth control. We will be more interested here with just looking at a few of the particulars with a focus on obtaining the results of the lab work to review in the next section. Even though, you will have your blood drawn at the end of week 4, you will not necessarily receive the results until possibly 1-2 weeks later. So we will hold off on our in depth discussion of the results until the next section (Weeks 5-12). For now, as a reminder, when you go in for all your blood labs, be sure to ask for a copy of all the results. What we will be looking at more closely in the next section are the hemoglobin (Hgb), white blood count (WBC), and absolute neutrophil count (ANC).

Section References

1. Viral kinetics in HCV
http://www.rcplondon.ac.uk/pubs/journal/journ_34_sep_conf3.htm *Dr G R Foster, Imperial College School of Medicine at St Mary's, London*

2. Hoefs, J.C., Morgan, T.R., *Seventy-two weeks of peginterferon and ribavirin for patients with partial early virologic response?*, Hepatology, 2007, Dec;46(6):1671-4

7

Weeks 5-12

Izabella's Story

It was April 3, 2009 and the day was a typical hectic rat race at work. For the last 8 months, I hadn't been feeling my usual self. Other than seeing a doctor 2 or 3 times a year for basic things I had always been pretty healthy with a lot of energy. I had seen a few doctors and wondered why none of them had ordered lab work. They all were attributing everything to menopause or age. Some of the symptoms were extreme fatigue, dizziness, nausea, very dry skin & hair and very unhealthy nails and cuticles. For nearly 8 months, my tongue and throat were inflamed. All my taste buds fell off my tongue and it was absolutely raw and looked like hamburger. It was so very painful, but none of the doctors knew what to do. I couldn't eat or drink anything with any real flavor or spices. It felt on fire all the time. I was miserable and new there was something wrong. There was!! After insisting on having my labs drawn by a new doctor I felt I would get some answers.

About a week later I was sitting at my desk when my doctor called me. I would usually get results by mail, so this was new. She said "Well it looks like you will have to stop drinking your wine because you have Hepatitis C." Straight and to the point I guess. Not sure what was worse, the diagnosis, or no wine? She stated that I would need to see a specialist & get a liver biopsy. Although I worked in a Lab, I actually knew very little about Hepatitis C. I just knew it must be something really bad. I guess you could say that once I heard this diagnosis, I shut my phone off and I just sat at my chair looking at my computer screen. Inside I was saying NO, this can't be real. My heart was pounding, ears were ringing and I just felt frozen in fear. Before I new it, I was just sobbing and sobbing. I remember sending text messages to my three boys with these words. "I guess my past has caught up to me." Each of them called me, and I gave them the news. I cried all day and was literally worthless at work. Learning more about this evil virus I took the frame of mind that I was going to die. I even wrote out my will and personal letters to my boys. I thought about my new grandson. Would I see him grow up? Frankly, I was in a daze. However upon searching the internet, I found the most wonderful and supportive website that gave me back not only HOPE, but through it all, became my second family. I could have never dealt with this without all of their caring hearts.

Since I work in a lab, I was able to get my results before my doctor. I had a viral load of 3.3 million, genotype 1b and this had been in my body for about 33 years. It all made sense to me then. The past had caught up with me. My doctor recommended a treatment for 48 weeks called "Interferon and Ribavirin." It is a form of Chemo & Ribavirin that we do ourselves at home; a combo of 5 Riba's a day and 1 injection of Interferon a week. At first, I then decided to take my chances and try the natural approach and a lot of prayer. Two months later, I decided to test the odds, and do the treatment. My ultra-sound showed a little shadowing in my liver area, but all the other organs were fine. My biopsy results stated I had stage 2 fibrosis and my liver damage was a low stage 3.

I had heard about the side affects and the possibility hair loss. That thought left me terrified alone. The list could range from not bad to horrible. I of course had the later. The first 3 weeks weren't too bad; a little achy but manageable. After that, was a whole new ball of wax. I hurt so bad every minute, I could barely walk very far without gasping for air. My WBC was at a critical level and my memory was toast! Doctor put me on Neupogen to boost my WBC up. That created more side affects. My mom has Alzheimer's and I now knew how she must feel. I felt like singing the song "If I only had a brain" from the Wizard of OZ. The depression hit pretty hard and this was the first time in my life I actually thought seriously of suicide. I couldn't rationalize or see logic and within 3 months I lost 17 lbs. My skin sagged due to loss of muscle and migraines were daily. I was always so very tired all I wanted to do was stay in bed. But I had to work, or at least look like it. I was on my support group website daily and was not only able to give others support and education on this disease, but I was over whelmed with love and support myself. There are not enough words to express my gratitude. They are "Angels from Heaven."

After being on treatment for 13 weeks, I was one of the unlucky one's and taken off. I had not responded to the treatment well at all. My viral load was still 147K where is should have been undetected. Then is when I lost about 65% of my hair. It was coming out in huge chunks. The sides of my head were all but bald and my hair was so damaged from the medicine that I just shaved it off. So here it has been 5 months since I stopped treatment. I have gained all the weight back, Have about 2" of hair growth and feel pretty good. I may do the new treatment coming in 2011, but right now, I am just blessed to have found this wonderful cyber family and enjoy life as much as I can.

iZi 2010

Settling into Treatment

So, you have been on treatment now for four full weeks. As mentioned before, this is the initial adjustment phase. During the previous four weeks you have been introduced to many of the bothersome and some of the not so bothersome side effects that will surely pop up from time to time as you progress through treatment. During my first 4 weeks, I thought I was going to be one of the lucky ones who did not have to deal with the rash associated with taking Ribavirin. I only had a couple little red marks on my lower back and upper chest. However, after week 4, these marks started to multiply, and within a few more weeks, I had a few larger areas where I had the "itchies" off and on. I loved to take the back of my nails and just run them over the spots lightly, being careful not to break any skin. My rash never was more than just a nuisance and a little unsightly.

You have most likely learned which over the counter medications work for you in helping to alleviate many of the side effects. Most have to deal with headaches, and some insomnia. Some people may be reacting more quickly or adversely to the Riba Rash, and have a prescriptive remedy. In the rest of this section, we are going to be looking at lab results from your week 4 blood workup and ongoing and new side effects. We will also look at the importance of taking Omega-3 and other vitamins based on clinical research relating to HCV patients who eliminate the virus. The results of that study show that there in an actual negative consequence to the body for clearing the HCV virus in some individuals. Finally, we will discuss week 12 blood workup and what will be looked at for those results.

Week Four Lab Work Results

In all likelihood, you did have some blood drawn on your 4 week follow up visit to your treating physician. Here we will look at some important key indicators of how your body is responding to the medications. Everyone responds to the medications differently, because of our naturally occurring differences physiologically and because there appear to be different strains of the virus, even within genotype, that act more resistant than others to the treatment. Some of the things that will want to be looked at as soon as possible will be the way your blood levels are responding to both the Ribavirin and the Pegylated Interferon. We now revisit Hgb, WBC, and ANC levels from your blood work and what consequences there might be for your particular levels.

As mentioned previously, the Hgb level is the red blood cell count. Hgb binds and carries oxygen through the body. The Hgb level is measured to determine one's level of anemia. The recommended dosing of Ribavirin for genotypes 1 and 4 is 1200mg/day for patients >= 75kg body weight and 1000mg/day for body weight < 75kg. The recommended dosing modifications for Ribavirin for low hgb for patients with no history of cardiac disease is to reduce the Ribavirin to 600 mg/day for Hgb levels < 10.0 g/dL and to discontinue Ribavirin if Hgb falls below 8.5 g/dL [2]. Your lab results should indicate your 4 week level and the normal range. If your Hgb is below 11 at this point, you should take a look at the adverse side effects and management section to prepare yourself for a discussion with your doctor.[1]

Significant anemia (Hgb<10 g/dL) has been observed in up to 9%-13% of patients undergoing combination therapy, while moderate anemia (Hgb<11 g/dL) has been observed in up to 30% of patients. Now, in a one study it was found that 36% of all patients who discontinued treatment did so due to anemia, and this amounted to a full 8.8% of all patients. So, you can see that anemia is a very serious threat to winning the battle and achieving SVR. There are actually many options to dealing with anemia without the need for discontinuing treatment; please read up on them in the adverse side effects and management section now, so you can be prepared if and when you need to have a discussion with your doctor about your Hgb level.[2]

Some of the symptoms you are likely to experience from the Ribavirin present themselves as a feeling of becoming short of breath very easily, light headedness, and dizziness. The more pronounced these side effects are usually indicates the degree of anemia you may have, but not always. It is very likely that your quality of life will be affected by any anemia you may be experiencing. Many people who have undergone treatment have reported that even doing common household chores that used to be simply mundane but easily managed, now become more of a major undertaking. While some even have to resort to taking time off from work, at least on occasion, and although rarely, sometimes for the duration of treatment; many others still perform their employment activities, but upon returning home from work, most find that the remainder of the day is mostly spent resting either in bed or in a comfortable chair or couch. The psychological impact of this can be overwhelming at times, as one becomes very frustrated at the inability to maintain a normal lifestyle.

Your White Blood Count (WBC) and Absolute Neutrophil Count (ANC) are important indicators on how your body is responding. Absolute neutrophil count is the real number of white blood cells that are neutrophils. The normal range for the Absolute Neutrophil Count is 1.5 to 8.0 (1,500 to 8,000/mm3). The ANC is not measured directly, but is calculated by multiplying the WBC count times the percent of neutrophils in the differential WBC. The percent of neutrophils consists of the segmented neutrophils and the bands that are almost mature neutrophils.
Sample calculation of the ANC:

WBC count: 6,000 cells/mm3 of blood
Segs: 30% of the WBCs
Bands: 3% of the WBCs
Neutrophils (segs + bands): 33% of the WBCs
ANC: 33% X 6,000 = 2,000/mm3 ANC of 2,000/mm3, by convention = 2.0 Normal range: 1.5 to 8.0 (1,500 to 8,000/mm3)
Interpretation: Normal[3]

Neutropenia is a condition that makes a person vulnerable to infection. Neutrophils are key components in the system of defense against infection. An absence or scarcity of can lead to neutropenia. Chemotherapy, radiation, or a blood or marrow transplant can lead to a suppression of neutrophils, but afterward the ANC slowly rises, reflecting the fact that the bone marrow is recovering allowing new blood cells to grow and mature. In practical clinical terms, a normal ANC is 1.5 or higher; a "safe" ANC is 0.5 to 1.5; a low ANC is less than 0.5. A safe ANC usually means that the patient's activities do not need to be restricted (on the basis of the ANC alone).[3]

Ongoing and New Side Effects

Well by now, you have probably encountered most of the common, less serious, side effects by now. With your doctor's approval, you most likely have a solution for dealing with most of these, either with over the counter, home remedies, or with prescribed medications. Many patients, but not all, are either taking medications for headaches, nausea, insomnia, or depression that does occurs in a small, but significant, percentage of patients. One symptom we hear over and over that continues to frustrate is that of the Riba Rash. Because of this, we are going to discuss it in more detail now. Riba Rash usually does not cause one to have to discontinue or modify treatment, but in a small percentage it does. Here we will discuss common solutions to dealing with the rash, but for more serious reactions, please refer to the adverse side effects and management section for more in-depth information about solutions and of course, always consult your doctor about any and all side effects you experience while on or off treatment.

These methods for dealing with "Riba Rash" are taken from real life experiences from patients who have undergone treatment and experienced the rash first hand. Here we share with you their solutions. Steroid creams or ointments may help but need to be prescribed and monitored by your doctor as there can be side effects from long term use.

Here is a list of things recommended by a patient who underwent treatment that seem to help keep their skin in as good a shape as possible4

1. Shower or bathe no more than once daily.
2. Avoid hot water: this dries the skin out.
3. Use only Dove, Cetaphil, Purpose, or Vanicream soap, and use it sparingly.
4. Use a soft cotton washcloth or your hands to cleanse the skin. No not use rough sponges, loofas or buff puffs.
5. After showering, pat dry rather than rubbing.
6. Moisturize your skin immediately after each bath or shower (while the skin is still damp) with one of the creams/ointments listed below (creams or ointments work better than lotions)
7. Do not use perfumes or colognes.
8. Do not scratch or rub your skin.
9. Trim your nails short so that you don't accidentally scratch during your sleep.
10. Wear soft, non-binding cotton clothing and other natural fiber clothing.
11. Wash your clothes using Cheer Free, Tide Free or All Free & Clear.
12. Set your washer for an extra rinse cycle.
13. Do not use fabric softeners or dryer sheets.

Moisturizing Ointments and Creams:

1. Vanicream
2. Vaseline Petroleum Jelly (fragrance free)
3. White Petrolatum
4. Aquaphor
5. Cetaphil cream
6. Eucerin cream

Omega-3 and Other Cholesterol Improving Agents

Hopefully, you have been taking, at the very least, a multi-vitamin and doctor approved Vitamin-D supplements since even before taking that first shot. The benefits of Vitamin-D were outlined before, and of course, a multi-vitamin will help you keep your body physically fit, nutritionally speaking. We are now going to look at Omega-3 supplements and why it may be very important to also be taking this supplement during and after the course of treatment. Kathleen Corey and colleagues from Massachusetts General Hospital conducted a study to determine the rate of significant hyperlipidemia (high blood fat content) in HCV treated patients compared against a control group who had no HCV present in their blood. For the baseline, or control basis, the researchers first compared 179 HCV positive patients against 180 age-matched negative HCV control individuals for LDL (bad cholesterol), HDL (good cholesterol), and triglyceride levels.

Next they performed a retrospective cohort analysis on 87 patients who had been treated for HCV who had lipid values available for both before and after treatment. The results are very surprising and have very meaningful and medically relevant implications for the ongoing health impact on those successfully treated for HCV. The following is a list of key findings whose results remained consistent even after adjusting for sex, age, and HCV genotype:

1. In the case-control analysis, the HCV infected group had significantly lower LDL and total cholesterol levels than the uninfected control group.
2. In the retrospective cohort, Hepatitis C patients in the treated group who achieved virological response, or HCV clearance, had larger increases in LDL and total cholesterol from baseline than patients without viral clearance.
3. 13% of patients with virological clearance had elevated LDL levels and 33% had elevated total cholesterol levels that warranted lipid-lowering therapy.

The authors of the study concluded that being infected with Hepatitis C is associated with lower cholesterol levels and in particular, a lower LDL than those not infected with the virus. What this means is that the virus itself is providing a beneficial effect on the body in terms of "bad cholesterol" by reducing the LDL levels in those infected. They also concluded that a significant percentage of HCV patients successfully treated experience a rebound in total cholesterol levels and LDL to levels associated with a higher risk for coronary, or heart, disease. Based on their findings, they recommend monitoring and assessing cholesterol levels in patients who are successfully treated for HCV as a follow up care procedure, as achieving clearance of the virus may reveal individuals with previously unidentifiable coronary risk.[5]

Remarkably, it looks like having HCV may help keep in check cholesterol levels, but after successful treatment, a previously unidentified risk may now exhibit itself. Well, knowing this information is really good, because it means we can start to do something now to help reduce the chance of this threat from occurring. By taking action early on in the treatment process, we can help our bodies by doing some things that will help offset the lost beneficial effect on cholesterol that results from viral clearance. Prior to treatment, I was taking some fish oil supplements, because my doctor had suggested this after some of my cholesterol levels were shown to be a bit high. During treatment, I sort of slacked off on some of my vitamins and supplements, but after I found an article describing the results just mentioned, I immediately started my good regimen of vitamins and supplements I had been following prior to treatment. The following is a list of things one can do to help bring down one's "bad cholesterol" and raise one's "good cholesterol."

To help raise HDL, or one's good cholesterol try one or more of the following:

1. Quit Smoking, which can dramatically improve HDL.
2. Start a regular exercise routine.
3. Maintain a healthy weight.
4. Abstain from drinking alcohol during treatment, even though moderate use of alcohol can raise one's HDL.
5. Eating more monosaturated fat found in olive and other vegetable oils, nuts (for the non-allergic people), and avocados can help raise HDL while at the same time help reduce LDL and triglycerides. This should result in a lower risk of heart disease.

6. Take daily Omega-3 supplements. People who took one gram of an Omega-3 fatty acid supplement reduced their risk of a sudden cardiac death by 42 percent.

One of the main purposes of this book it to maximize one's chance of achieving SVR, while at the same time doing what is necessary to get through and survive the treatment process. Surviving treatment also means doing what we can to counter any negative results that might arise from clearing this virus from our body. Let's start now and do what is necessary, so that we come through the other side and maximize our chances of having healthy cholesterol levels.

Week 12 Blood Tests

The 12 week marker the usual blood tests include: CBC w/diff (complete blood count with differential), LFT (liver function test), TSH (thyroid), HCV RNA quantitative (viral count). It will be very important to learn the viral load results from the 12 week treatment mark. We will discuss this in a bit more depth in the next section.

Section References

1.
http://www.gene.com/gene/products/information/pegasys/pdf/Copegus_pi.pdf

2. 1: Ong JP, Younossi ZM. Managing the hematologic side effects of antiviral therapy for chronic Hepatitis C: anemia, neutropenia, and thrombocytopenia. Cleve Clin J Med. 2004 May;71 Suppl 3:S17-21. Review. PubMed PMID: 15468613.

3. http://www.medterms.com/script/main/art.asp?articlekey=20030

4. http://hcvsupport.org/forum/index.php/topic,3229.0.html

5. K Corey, E Kane E, C Munroe, and others. Hepatitis C virus infection and its clearance alter circulating lipids: implications for long-term follow-up. *Hepatology*. 50(4): 1030-1037. October 2009.

8

Weeks 13-24

Terri O's Story

The day I found out I was positive for HCV started out full of potential and excitement! After the birth of our first child, I experienced 3 miscarriages over the next year. My husband and I had been referred to a fertility clinic, and after initial standard testing I went in for one last procedure. Afterwards, the doctor said she needed to speak with me in her office. I figured we were going to discuss test results and set up a timetable for IVF. All my fertility related tests came up normal. But I was positive for Hepatitis C. Just like that...full of hope, and then thrown into a world where I didn't know how to feel or what to think. I was blank. Emotionless. Expressionless. She said the next step was getting a viral load test done. Maybe I had been exposed but didn't actually have HCV.

I had the viral load test done that day. I had no idea that it would take two excruciatingly long weeks to get the results. I cried the whole time; I kept hoping that it was all some horrible mistake. I kept thinking, "but I'm healthy!" I never had any health problems, and didn't have any of the risk factors I found listed that would predispose me to contracting HCV. "It had to be a false positive, there is no other possibility," I thought. Two weeks later I got the call: my viral load was over 5 million. I returned to my gynecologist, who up until that point had been the only doctor I needed. I have known her for years, everyone was sympathetic, and fortunately the nurse took me aside and gave me sound advice: go to a general practitioner for a referral, but find a good specialist. "Most doctors won't know much about what you are going to go through," she said, "research and find someone who knows what they are doing."

My new general practitioner ordered a liver ultrasound, more liver enzyme tests, and a genotype test. Waiting for referrals, and test results gave me time to research and learn a lot. I stopped drinking wine, though I only had a glass or two a week prior to my diagnosis. I started focusing on getting 5-9 servings of veggies a day, drinking a lot of fluids and generally being good to my body. I made it a point to get to the gym and work on building my stamina and muscle in anticipation of keeping fit through treatment. I had always followed a healthy lifestyle, but now it was my life!

My tests came back with normal ultrasound, liver enzymes had come down, and I was genotype 3. I released a big sigh of relief; genotype 3 would only mean 24 weeks of treatment, not 48. We could get back to trying to conceive within a year! Or so I thought...

One thing we get to do a lot of when diagnosed is wait. By the time I got in to see the specialist, 6 months had passed. Two more went by while I waited for a nurse to be available to monitor me. My viral load had gone down on it's own to 3 million by the time I started. I was told this is quite common; it ebbs and flows along with our immune response. Since I had genotype 3, my hepatologist didn't think a biopsy was necessary. I could have one if I wished, but he recommended a Fibrosure II test. My score was very low, indicating no fibrosis, so I decided against the biopsy.

I always worked on eating a healthful diet and doing regular workouts, and my hepatologist was pleased that I was starting off from such a good spot, it influences how well we respond to treatment. He recommended that I continue my workouts to the maximum level I could tolerate during treatment, especially light cardiovascular exercise, and lifting light weights to keep muscle tone intact. He said it would lessen side effects, help me maintain my weight and muscle, and ultimately make recovery faster and easier.

Treatment has been a whirlwind of good and bad days. Mostly good, though the definition of good has changed from my pre treatment, lively self! A good day means my side effects are controlled with some ibuprofen or acetaminophen, and I have enough energy to do most of the things I need to. Rest is important, but so is getting the exercise I need. I found that a light workout helped my mental outlook, and gave me more of the energy I needed to keep going. Nutrition was difficult. My appetite was lacking, but if I didn't eat (or ate poorly) it really affected my energy levels. I took to adding pureed organic baby vegetables to my juices, and some of my main dishes to get them in. The antioxidants are so important to healing, but eating fresh vegetables (or smelling them cooking) was difficult. I tried to eat as many nutrient dense foods as I could in between protein shakes, and whatever I could stomach.

I just finished treatment this week! My virus has been undetectable since week two, so I am entirely optimistic that I will achieve SVR. I made it through with the support of my immediate family, and my online support group. Without all the friends who were going through the same things I was experiencing, I don't know if I could have worked through everything so well. My family was very supportive, but some things they can't understand. It hasn't been easy, but it was doable. I just had to take everything day by day.

Terri O

Week Twelve Lab Work Results

At the 12 week marker the usual blood tests include: CBC w/diff (complete blood count with differential), LFT (liver function test), TSH (thyroid), HCV RNA quantitative (viral count). The goal is to either have been found undetectable by this point or at least to have achieved a 2 log drop from your baseline viral load. If the viral load comes back undetected, then means you have achieved a "complete early viral response", or cEVR. Those who achieve either a Rapid Viral Response (RVR) or cEVR have a statistically higher chance for a successful treatment outcome, than those who do not fully clear the virus until after week 12. Please see the section on SVR Estimator for detailed information.

If you are a slower responder, then your goal is to achieve undetectable status before 24 wks. Those who do not have an undetectable viral load test result by week 24 are usually discontinued from any further treatment, as continuing has a very low likelihood of a successful outcome. Be sure to get a copy of any blood test results that you have performed at this stage of the treatment process, and file them away for safe-keeping. It will also be instructive to go over the results and compare them to your 4 week results with your doctor, and discuss how your doctor feels your treatment process is progressing in comparison to "typical" results.

The New "Normal"

Hopefully when you reach this point you have begun to develop a routine, and have had some idea of what side effects you might be encountering and how to handle them. The first 12 weeks can bring about such a myriad of symptoms. Anemia, shortness of breath, fatigue and lack of energy, headaches, rash, depression, irritability, anxiety, and lack of appetite may have come to visit you. They may have also become easily manageable or even subsided in some cases. However, if you're having symptoms that you can't manage, talk to your doctor or health care provider. Write down a list of issues you are concerned about and questions that are nagging at you and take them to your next appointment. Never hesitate to call your doctor immediately if you have questions or concerns that are of a pressing nature. Reaction to treatment is quite individual; no one reacts or responds the same way to treatment. Management of HCV has been studied long enough to know the most common side effects of treatment medications and how to best treat the individual.

A word of caution at this part of your journey – don't give up. You may feel worse than you've ever felt, and it may feel like it won't end. Just as HCV is a chronic disease that lasts a lifetime, unless you successfully treat it, HCV treatment can seem just as chronic with its longevity of treatment. But this is finite, usually only lasting 24 weeks or 48 weeks, depending on genotype and early response to treatment. If we are to have a chance at achieving an SVR, we must first survive the treatment process. In order to do that, we must learn to live this new lifestyle that has been thrust upon us, by the treatment process. Many of us who have undergone treatment and who are currently undergoing treatment as of this writing refer to this new lifestyle as the "new normal." Our day to day activities have become quite different (unless you are in the group who experience little or no side effects). However, if we can incorporate some good healthy habits into this new lifestyle, it will go a long way to ensuring we are able to get through each day and the one after that until completion. Let's discuss some of these lifestyle habits that might point toward achieving a continued successful completion of treatment.

Diet

Continue to drink lots of water. It's essential to prevent dehydration as this could lead to a worsening of symptoms. Caffeine can contribute to water loss, so it's best to use it in moderation, and stay away from it in the evening as this could exacerbate any symptoms of insomnia you may be having. If you like the power drinks, find the ones that have the least sugar, caffeine and fat content. The liver metabolizes fat, and when a person consumes too much fat, the liver has difficulty metabolizing it completely. Then it becomes stored in the liver. Your liver doesn't like that either.

It's very important to eat a well-balanced diet, with fresh fruits and vegetables. You may be having trouble with side effects which interfere with adequate nutritional intake. Those can include nausea, indigestion, sore tongue or mouth, but again, this is treatable. Find those "comfort" foods that don't increase symptoms. It is also very important to eat with the Ribavirin. Many have found that if they take the Ribavirin on an empty stomach and forget to eat, they experience nausea. Food helps this, even if it's just ice cream, my personal favorite for the evening dose.

One study, carried out on a large number of HCV patients and controls, demonstrated that dietary intake affects liver histology, and indirectly, response to treatment. In fact, a univariate and multivariate analysis showed that a high intake of calories, carbohydrates, and lipids was associated with more severe fibrosis. Weight reduction has been shown to reduce steatosis (fatty liver disease), abnormal liver enzymes, and improve fibrosis in patients with chronic Hepatitis C. This finding illustrates that diet is an important factor in the management of patients affected by HCV.

Exercise

You may not feel like "working out." Or, you may not be able to "work-out" like you once did. But do what you can. Prevent atrophy of those muscles or muscle wasting. As often and as much as you can tolerate, do some sort of physical exercise. If you are anemic, even the smallest amount of exertion can lead to shortness of breath and rapid heart rate. So use common sense, don't over do. Consider that you have been given a bucket full of energy. How you use it, is up to you. How fast it fills back up is the new story while in treatment. Monitor what your response to activity is, and if you over-do one day, you may have to rest more the following day. The other benefit of exercise is it normalizes your life. There have been multiple studies done on the psychological benefits of exercise. Personally, cleaning the bathroom has become my work out for the day. Plan your projects and how you'll spend your bucket of energy. Spread them out if possible.

Boredom and Doldrums

Welcome to the roller coaster. As you move through the weeks, you may find them meshing into one another and you measure success as more good days than bad. Especially when you've got symptoms managed, it becomes a journey through the day punctuated by medications at the minimum of every 12 hours. It's very important not to forget any. Your energy has dwindled and you may have cut a lot of personal activities that give you pleasure. Your battery isn't being recharged. You may experience a sense of loss and grief for the things in life that give you the most pleasure as it becomes an everyday treatment, treatment, treatment; what sides will I have today? What will I be able to do?

It will be difficult to make plans. You may say, "I don't have the energy to do anything and if I do, then I feel worse." Let it be stressed here, that this can change week to week. Many have very good days punctuated by the occasional bad days. Others seem to have good weeks and bad weeks. During my 24 week course of treatment, I had two separate full weeks where I almost felt completely normal. I also had three full separate weeks where I felt like I had the flu; I may actually have had the flu on one of those occasions, but it is very hard to differentiate the normal treatment side effects from flu like symptoms, so that is a mystery that will never be answered. The other weeks were somewhere in between those two extremes, and this sort of roller coaster ride of side effects seems to be what is reported most by those who have communicated with on this issue.

As your energy level has now most likely plummeted to an all time low, you may find yourself experiencing a day to day life that is very boring and full of drudgery much of the time. Many people find activities to keep them out of this funk. Preparing healthy foods that are not only good for you, but are compatible with any mouth or appetite side effects is a very good method to use. Exercise, while perhaps now much more moderated, is also a very healthy way to not only keep busy, but help maintain as much muscle mass as possible during treatment. Getting out to the gym will be a low priority for most, but using indoor exercise equipment can be a suitable alternative. To sum up, you should now be a veteran at the HCV treatment experience.

If you have made it this far, you are actually probably done if you are genotype 2 or 3, or have possibly been on a trial study with some of the new medications now being tested in clinical trials. However, if you are like the majority, you are on standard of care and belong to the genotype 1 group who are treating for a full 48 weeks. If that is the case, don't fret, because if you have made it this far, and your 24 week viral load shows undetected, and you continue on to another 24 weeks of treatment, it will most likely feel like you are just going through the routine day after day. You now know how to deal with issues as they arise, and have a routine for getting through each day. Even though you may test as undetected now, more treatment is necessary to try to eliminate every single last HCV virus that may be "hiding" out in various parts of the body. If that happens, you will test negative for HCV at 6 months post treatment and be deemed SVR, and in effect be cured.

Week 24 Blood Tests

The end of week 24 marks another important milestone. You may be discontinuing treatment because you are genotype 2 or 3 or because you were unable to clear the virus by 24 weeks of treatment. If you are undetected and classified as genotype 1 or 4, you are most likely continuing on for another 24 weeks of treatment. So continue with the next section if you are continuing treatment; however if you are stopping now, please skip to the "Post Treatment Recovery" section.

9

Weeks 25-48

MagickBalls' Story

If you are reading this, I imagine it's because you have recently been diagnosed with Hepatitis C, or you have a loved one, or a good friend you care about that has. A nasty disease that can take a life, if left to go it's natural course. Our friends in the medical community have given us a treatment that can work. Not everyone completes it. Not everyone gets positive results; meaning it's consistently found undetectable in your body. For others, it happens, and so far I count myself as one of those lucky individuals. Here's my story.

During the Spring of 2008, I found out I had Hepatitis C. Responding to an ad needing people with acid reflux for a study. Have done this a few times over the years in the past. Earn a little extra money, and help drug companies come up with new ways to treat what I routinely suffered with; Win-Win situation. I went in, and interviewed. They did a regular check up, taking some blood in the process. Doctor called me with results some days later. I tested positive for Hepatitis C. Said I should go to my regular Doctor to confirm; did that. Results also came in positive; Genotype: 1a / Viral Count: 5.5 million.

Can't be sure how I got it. Many possibilities:

1. *My Mom had Hepatitis when I was born.*
2. *I have two tattoos. Got one in 1980. Another in 1992*
3. *Working in a hospital in the late 70's doing general clean up, I got poked on two different occasions with dirty needles that were placed in the trash, instead of the proper place where they should have been disposed of.*
4. *Was a teenager in the 70's. Worked hard. Played hard. I partied, and continued to do so, into the 80's. Sometimes excessively. Can't say being consistent using the best judgment applied here. Drinking heavily, doing occasional drugs, and having sex with girls you just met isn't exactly what the Surgeon General recommends to maintaining a healthy lifestyle.*

Focusing on this ended up a waste of time. Most important fact was that I had it. Came to terms with the diagnosis, and proceeded to go from there. Told my wife. I really had no solid answers but the fact was I had it. Forty seven years old at the time. In good shape for the most part. Bloated stomach. Sometimes fatigued. Suffering pains in my legs. The last few years. Yet my yearly physical always came back fine. Now Doctors were answering questions for me. I was spending time researching on the Internet. Odds are I had this condition for many years.

Speaking of Doctors, I lost interest in the one who was going to treat me, and found one I liked better. Glad I did. Treatment is 48 weeks. Having a good relationship with your physician is vital. This Doctor had my wife and I attend a class before I started taking the prescribed medication. Combined treatment 101. A good time was had by all. Mentioning my wife, she tested negative for Hepatitis C. Married almost 15 years now. Dated a year and a half before we put the rings on. Had all the sex two normal people could have during that period. I was worried. Way more for her then I was myself. Grateful she didn't have it.

Treatment consisted of taking pills twice a day, and giving yourself a needle once a week. The needle part freaked me out. In the stomach or thighs. I told myself there was no way I could administer a shot to myself. Period! My wife did the first ones. Then she was admitted in the hospital. Complications from heart surgery she recently had. Came time I had to do the shot myself. Frightened to death, I did so. It was too important to my wife and myself. Successful treatment meant I could possibility live a longer, healthier life. Looking back, I find it amazing that I not only alone at home, did that shot, but also did every other shot after that. Hated it each and every time.

Next came the side effects. Almost immediately I suffered from cold and flu symptoms. Coughing and having a runny nose was everyday, for the entire time. Imagine having a cold for almost a year. Unbelievable. Damn near unbearable at times. Here's when I learned about rescue medication. Mostly over the counter drugs that would help with whatever ailment you were suffering with at the time. My new habit was sucking on cough drops. Throughout combined treatment, regular cold and flu medicine helped as   well.

I worked my whole time during the 48 week course. Missed one day due to stomach problems; violent crapping. How *dramatic. Can you say, diarrhea? I drive, doing locals deliveries for a auto parts store, for a living. Not doing treatment, one bad meal at a Mexican fast food place could render a person with this anyway. Driving and diarrhea don't mix. Waking up to this unpleasant surprise, I called out for the day.*

During the big pig flu outbreak of 2009, there I was at my employment, coughing, and sneezing every day. Yet I wasn't sick. No cold. Co-workers will wonder after a while. Many doing the same treatment, take time off from work. It's understandable. Some people suffer from side effects way worse than I did. Some do the treatment, and it doesn't work for them. I feel so bad for them. I can't imagine going through all this, and it not having any positive rewards.

I told three people I had Hep C. To everyone else I had a cold. Just not feeling well that day. Excuse works for people who are not around you everyday. Back to my co-workers. I didn't feel obligated to disclose to my job that I had Hepatitis C. Fact is in part, due to stupid late night comedians, and folks totally ignorant on the subject, the information about how one acquires such a disease is negative, and not necessarily true. Not that unprotected sex with anything that breathes, or being a intravenous-drug addict is a bad thing. But not something I wanted my co-workers, or for that fact, other folks in my family, or even acquaintances to believe about me. I personally feel that it's up to the individual as to how vocal they are with others about what they are suffering from. I decided it was best for me, not wearing it on my sleeve. Still, how can one have a cold for 48 weeks? A white lie did the trick. Said I was being treated for ulcers. Strong medicine that had side effects. Will keep being a great excuse until the day one of them comes across this book, reads it, and figures out they been had.

Back to side effects. What's worse, anemia or the consistent cold & flu symptoms, I've experienced since doing treatment? Answer, they both sucked through a long straw. Add to that the brain fog. Vision being sensitive. Hearing loss. Lack of appetite. I lost 40 pounds. Fifty percent of the food that went in my mouth, tasted like metal. Twenty five percent, like dirt. And the last twenty five percent, not as good as it should taste. Sex life went pretty much down the toilet. Had periods of rage, that I was lucky enough to keep a handle on. Some bruising from the shots. Itching / rash. Hair falling out. Awkwardness being around people because of coughing / generally not feeling well. Lack of energy. At least two days a week of stomach problems; annoying pains / diarrhea. When they told me here was a list of possible side effects caused from combined treatment, I didn't think I would get most of them. Luck of the Irish, but I handled it. Some days that was very hard. My day might have consisted of working, and then heading right to bed when I came home. Survived. One day turned into a week, that turned into a month, that came over time, 48 solid weeks. Never did think I would finish, but I did. Plain and simple hanging in there, helped accomplish that. Took my medicine when I was suppose to, and grinned and beared the rest.

Speaking of luck, blood tests showed since week 6 of treatment that I've been undetectable. Worth putting up, dealing with the side effects from the medication? In my opinion; of course. Anything that can make you live a better, longer quality life is. Here's a screw in the works.

About half way through treatment, my appendix decided it was time to leave. Was taken off both meds for ten days. Till I had my staples taken out. Was worried a break in treatment might cause negative results. It was cool. Still undetectable.

Have now finished treatment, on New Years Eve of 2009. Takes time for the two medicines to clear your system totally. I was advised it would be 3 to 6 months before I started feeling like my old self. Over three weeks into this I can say they were not kidding me when they said that. Slowly I'm coming back. Food tastes better. My penis appears to be coming out of it's long slumber. Happy days ahead for sure.

The road has been traveled before. Some make the journey, and some crash. Don't be afraid. Do what your Doctor recommends. You won't be their first patient with Hepatitis C. Maybe find others going through the same thing; Internet. Strength in numbers. And tell yourself no matter what, you can do this.

My experience. My opinions. My observations. Thanks for reading. Whatever your situation is, good luck.

Started Treatment: 01/17/09. Viral Count 4 weeks into treatment: 197. Around my 6th week; UNDETECTABLE. Last shot (Pegasys 180 MCG / 0.5ML); 12/26/09. Finished pills; Ribavirin 600 MG - twice a day on 12/31/09.

Anonymous 48 year old male from Houston, TX., U.S.A.

Reaching the Summit and Renewing Your Resolve

Well, if you are reading this section, then that most likely means you are continuing treatment for a full 48 weeks. As of this writing, you can count yourself among the majority. Until a 24 week treatment regimen is approved for genotype 1, the standard of care treatment is usually a full 48 weeks. One outstanding thing about finding yourself at this stage of treatment is that being here means you have been able to muster through the first 24 weeks without either being dropped from treatment for a lack of proper response, dropped out due to being unable to manage any adverse side effects that might have occurred, or dropped out due to the inability to cope with all that treatment brings upon oneself. You should still have an undetected viral load and are most likely now very adjusted to treatment and your new "normal" lifestyle. You know how to deal with and manage your side effects, and you have hopefully developed some good habits in the areas of diet and exercise. As well, you should have a very good support system in place.

This is the march through the weeks. You are at the halfway mark, a major milestone. From here on out, instead of counting the weeks already completed, you can start counting down the weeks left. You may at times get overwhelmed. You will see others who have genotype 2 and 3 completing treatment and getting to stop at this 24 week mark. To have to go through treatment for HCV is a grueling ordeal. We should all feel fortunate there is a treatment that often results in successful eradication. Even to have to go through 24 weeks is a life altering thing. Let us at this time realize we have done the hardest 24 weeks already, renew our resolve, and continue on to the finish line, where it will be our turn to dance in triumphant jubilation. Then we can return to our normal lives; return to our family and loved ones, who have surely felt nothing but empathy and concern while suffering alongside us through this treatment ordeal.

Now, for the next 24 weeks, there isn't much more we can offer in terms of trying to prepare you on how to maximize your chances for success or to survive treatment. However, one reason that some of those who go through treatment and either have a viral breakthrough during treatment (where the virus returns before the end of treatment) or have a viral relapse (where the virus returns after the completion of treatment) is due to non-compliance to taking the medications at the dosages or frequency prescribed. Skipping doses or taking lower doses than prescribed can be very risky in terms of allowing the virus to break through or survive the treatment process. Once the virus is undetectable in the blood, it usually takes awhile longer to actually eradicate the virus from the blood; this is due to the fact that the viral load tests can only detect virus down to a certain threshold level; one of the more sensitive tests still can only detect concentrations down to about 15 copies per milliliter. Also, even after the virus is completely gone from the blood, the medications are still "finding" and destroying virus in other parts of the body where the virus may be "hiding" out. This is why treatment must continue for some time even after one is deemed to have undetectable virus in their blood.

Let us remind you of this; there is nothing better to get you through the boredom and doldrums than having a good support system in place. No one really knows what it is like to go through treatment except those who have or are currently undergoing the same treatment. This is where online support forums, such as the companion one for this book, www.hcvshare.org can help you in dealing with the every day issues that arise relating to treatment. To make sure you have someone you can communicate with who really understands and can offer solutions that have been tried and proven, please find yourself either a local support group or an online forum or both. Not only will you be able to get support from those in a similar situation as yourself, but you will be able to give support to others as well. Together, you and your support group will be able to get through the final phase of your treatment, and rejoice together as it comes to a close. After treatment is completed, there will a recovery phase; the medications do not leave your body overnight once you stop taking them. The next section is dedicated to what comes after treatment.

10

Post Treatment Recovery

Larry M's Story

I found out that I had HCV as the result of a complete physical exam in the year in 2000. I had been a heroin IV drug user for the years between 1976 and 1981. In 1982 I went on methadone maintenance to treat me for my heroin addiction. In 1986 I was introduced to 12 step recovery, and have been drug & alcohol free ever since. It has been a great life of freedom and hope to be free of those demons of my past.

When I found out I had HCV, I was happily married for 10 years, had a 4 year old boy, and my wife was expecting a baby girl any day. My initial feeling was that my life was over and I had been assigned a death sentence at the age of 45. I felt scared, and was living in fear. Luckily, I had friends in recovery from substance abuse who had been down this path. They told me to get a liver biopsy and educate myself on this disease. Being proactive made me feel like I was involved in the solution, not the problem. I got my first liver biopsy about a month after being diagnosed. My liver damage was only at stage 1. My viral load was only about 750,000. I believe the reason my liver was in such good shape is because I had not had any alcohol or drugs for 15 years.

At that time, with the minimal liver damage, and Pegylated interferon still in trials, my doctor recommended that I get a biopsy every 5 years to monitor the liver. I had another biopsy in 2005, and the liver damage was still at stage 1. No further damage. In 2008, my energy levels were terrible, and if I didn't get 8 hours sleep, I would get a migraine headache, and I felt generally lousy for a guy who was in excellent physical shape and lived a healthy lifestyle. I went to my General Practitioner, and he recommended another biopsy. Long story short, my liver damage had gone from a stage 1 to stage 2-3 in 4 years!

My liver doctor happened to be involved in HCV drug trials. He said there were new drugs, that when used in combination with Interferon and Ribavirin, could knock out the virus in 6 months! This is an excellent prognosis for a guy with HCV genotype 1! He recommended that I join a trial with an experimental Protease Inhibitor, in combination with the current standard of care therapy that he was conducting. I started treatment in September 2009. My Viral load started at 4.5 million. Within two weeks, it had been reduced to 254, and after 1 month, the virus was Undetectable! These were the results that they were looking for. I continued to stay undetectable through all 24 weeks of treatment. My treatment ended on February 17, 2010.

I am now recovering from the rigors of treatment. I had become anemic as the result of the Ribavirin, so my body is weak. I feel a lot of hope that I will remain HCV free. I will

*continue with the trial, and they will be monitoring my
viral load for the next year.*

Larry

Post treatment Side Effects

Both Pegasys and Ribavirin will stay in your body for a
certain amount of time even after one has completed
treatment and is no longer taking the medications. So,
we can expect to continue to experience side effects from
both medications (and any other medications we were or
are still taking) for some time. Pegasys has a half-life of
50-80 hours.[1] A little over 14 days after last Pegasys shot,
there would still be 5% of the Pegasys remaining in your
system, according to the stated half-life. So, we can
expect very little Pegasys to be remaining after only a few
weeks, however, Ribavirin has a much longer half-life.

The mean steady-state γ-phase half-life of Ribavirin in
380 patients treated with peginterferon-α-2a plus
Ribavirin was 303 h, which was predicted to be achieved
after 7-11 weeks of treatment (4-6 half-lives of
Ribavirin)[2]. This means that it takes 7-11 weeks for the
body to become saturated with Ribavirin and to reach a
constant concentration in the body. The half life is about
12.6 days. Accordingly, even after a complete month of
discontinuing the Ribavirin, there is still about 10% of the
steady-state concentration in the body. Even months
later, there can still be traces of it in the body; this is the
main reason it is necessary to remain on two separate
forms of birth control and to be tested for pregnancy up to
six months following discontinuation of treatment.

Given this information about how long it takes to completely remove the medications from our system, we need to be aware of the fact that we will continue to experience side effects for some time after completing treatment. The time this occurs and the intensity to which the side effects remain varies somewhat from individual to individual. While most seem to indicate getting back to normal after only a few short weeks, a few seem to experience some of the side effects for more extended periods of time, even as far out as six months to a year after completing treatment. Others have been taking anti-depressants during treatment and the decision to stop or taper off these meds, as well as other meds taken to help combat side effects, should be discussed in depth with your treating doctor.

Post Treatment Viral Load Tests

Normally you will have an HCV RNA test for viral load at week 48, to confirm the virus is still undetectable, and at week 72 to test whether you have achieved a sustained viral response, defined as a negative test for HCV RNA 6 months post treatment (SVR). Some individuals may have viral load tests in between these times, and the closer you are to the magical 6 month mark and still come up undetectable, the more confident one can be that the 6 month mark will also come up undetectable. Most who do have a viral relapse (virus once again becomes detectable in the blood stream) do so in the first few weeks after ending treatment. Long term studies have shown a very small percentage of people who have achieved an SVR response testing positive again after the 6 month period, however, these few individuals who tested positive could not be ruled out as having been re-infected. Indeed, while you probably never hear a doctor declaring someone who has achieved SVR status as "cured", it is generally accepted that once SVR is achieved, the likelihood of somehow becoming positive for HCV RNA in the blood stream later on from spontaneous re-emergence is somewhat miniscule.

Returning to Normal Life

Keeping and maintaining healthy behaviors and lifestyle that were assumed during treatment should be a priority goal. The past 24, 48, or possibly even more, weeks of treatment have no doubt taken a toll on ones body and mind. Prior to and during treatment, if you have been following our guidelines and suggestions, you should have either maintained very good lifestyle habits or developed some new ones. Indeed it is many of these behavioral changes that enable one to maximize their chances of conquering the virus while at the same time surviving the treatment process. Coming through, we will now want to celebrate our new found freedom by doing what is right for our bodies, minds, and spirits; maintaining a very good healthy lifestyle is one of the best ways possible to accomplish this.

Even though we may have gone through the treatment process and have a good chance at remaining virus free, this does not mean that we are now immune to contracting the virus again through re-infection by one of the transmission modes. Those of us infected by HCV all contracted the virus by some means. For many, it may have been from a tattoo received many years prior to being diagnosed, for others it may have been from old IV illicit drug use, and for others it might have been from accidentally being exposed while working in the health care industry. There are a myriad of methods by which one can get exposed. Since we are not immune, we are still susceptible to re-infection by either the same genotype as before or by one of the other genotypes. Let's do what we can to not have to go through this treatment process yet another time, shall we?

Points to Remember

1. The side effects of treatment will continue for some time, even after the end of treatment.
2. Becoming pregnant must be avoided, not only during treatment, but for the first 6 months following discontinuation of treatment.
3. SVR is defined as negative HCV RNA test 6 months following treatment.
4. You should strive to maintain your good healthy habits developed prior to and during treatment, even after treatment ends.
5. Even though you may achieve SVR status, you can become re-infected, just as any other person can. You do NOT become immune just because you have been successfully treated for Hepatitis C.

Section References

1. http://www.janis7hepc.com/differences_between_pegasys_and.htm

2. Wade JR, Snoeck E, Duff F, Lamb M, Jorga K. Pharmacokinetics of ribavirin in patients with Hepatitis C virus. *Br. J. Clin. Pharmacol.* 2006; 62: 710-14.

11

Adverse Side Effects and Management

Pegylated Interferon and Ribavirin are powerful medications used as the standard of care for HCV treatment. There can be side effects but let it be stressed here that each person reacts in there own unique way to treatment. Also, side effects wax and wane; side effects experienced one week may not be present the next week. Some people have a predisposition to specific side effects such as depression or migraine headaches and so a screening process should take place prior to treatment. Hydration is a critical factor in how one tolerates medication. A person should drink an ounce of water for every 2 pounds of their body weight. So if you weigh 150 lbs, you should try to drink 75 ounces of water per day. This is not meant to be an exhaustive look at the side effects of HCV treatment, but more of an overview of many. We may have left some out, so please always consult with your treating physician on all side effect issues. Now, let us look at some of the more common adverse side effects.

Fatigue

One of the most common side effects is fatigue. Fatigue plagues many people undergoing treatment and is difficult to cope with on an on going basis. Fatigue differs from being tired in that you wake up without any energy. It feels like you could be walking through sand or mud. A way to counteract fatigue is to get plenty of rest, but keep moving. Small amounts of exercise are beneficial, not only to your physical self but your mental and emotional well being. Don't overdo or you may find that your daily bucket of energy becomes depleted and is slow to re-fill.

Other frequent side effects experienced are muscle aches, headache and possibly fever. This is often caused by the interferon. It can also be described as flu-like symptoms. These symptoms are often worse in the beginning of treatment. They can be counter-acted by using some ibuprofen or acetaminophen prior to taking the injection. However, these symptoms may continue during the course of treatment. Drink plenty of water and use a mild over the counter pain reliever. No more than 2,000 milligrams of acetaminophen per day. As always though, get approval from your doctor for all over the counter medications and dosages you wish to consider using for side effect relief.

Rash

Ribavirin can cause a rash which can vary from mild to awful. Moisturizers and emollients on the skin are a wonderful asset to the drying properties of treatment. It helps prevent some rash from developing. Hot showers feel wonderful but can increase the drying of the skin, as does soap. This dryness can aggravate or help increase the severity of the rash. What ever you do, try not to scratch the itch. If the rash becomes too hard to manage, see your health care provider or a dermatologist. There are prescription medications available to help lessen the severity of the rash. Again, hydration is an important player in symptom management, so be sure to drink your daily recommended amount of water.

Hair Thinning

Hair thinning is caused by the interferon and is not dangerous but disturbing to the self-esteem, which may already be hammered by the meds. Don't wash your hair everyday, avoid blow dryers, hot curlers, irons, and be gentle to your scalp. Comb your hair gently. Once the treatment is over, any hair loss you may have experienced should grow back hair will grow again.

Appetite

Appetite problems include nausea, indigestion, and decreased appetite. Some people describe a metal taste in the mouth or food tasting odd. An important way to prevent problems is to take Ribavirin with food. Find foods that taste good and don't bother your digestion. Try eating small meals, frequently. Avoid foods that are spicy or extra-rich. Give yourself an edge by eating as healthy as possible. Smoothies pack a nutritional punch while being easy on the digestive system. A sore mouth or tongue can impact your ability to eat. Avoid acidic or spicy foods. Try rinsing your mouth with warm salt water. Try taking probiotics or eating yogurt. If none of these interventions help make sure you see your health care provider. You may need a prescription medication. It is not uncommon for a sore mouth to be caused by a yeast infection.

Mental Health

If you have a history of depression, suicidal ideation, substance abuse, or other psychiatric conditions, the HCV treatment medications can worsen these problems. It is very important that you speak with your health care provider regarding any history you may have with these problems and quite often; your health care provider may want you to begin some form of side effect management medication to stabilize your mood prior to beginning treatment for HCV. Even without a history of depression, Interferon is frequently the cause of depression, anxiety and/or irritability. Anti-depressants or anti-anxiety medication may be needed to minimize this particular side effect.

Do things you enjoy. Take care of what needs to be taken care of but avoid spreading yourself too thin. Your job is to beat the virus and get well while minimizing the effects of treatment so you can enjoy life as much as possible while you are combating this disease through treatment. I heard some very sage words that I would love to now share with you all:

"... Think about what you want to spend your time on. Do a pie chart in your mind of your time and decide where you really want to invest yourself. Your time is you, in a sense. So spend yourself on the things/people/activities you love. Take time for the things that enrich you spiritually. Of course extra time for rest is important. So is time for creative outlets that matter to you."

Get enough rest and sleep. Insomnia can tip a person over from being ok to being completely undone by many of the side effects, especially fatigue and depression. Avoid caffeine and too many liquids close to bedtime, and avoid eating too late as well. If you are unable to sleep, see your health care provider. Medications are available that you can try. Some over-the-counter preparations can worsen a dry mouth but can be very effective for helping with sleep. Therapy for any of these symptoms must be closely monitored and individualized by your health care provider. A phrase patients use when they are unable to focus or concentrate is "brain fog." This can be caused by any of the above symptoms which have just been discussed but also by inadequate fluid intake. People taking interferon and Ribavirin have to take in enough fluids, so drink your water!

Anemia

One of the serious side effects of Ribavirin is anemia, which is a low red blood count and can cause:

shortness of breath
rapid heart rate
weakness or fatigue
dose reduction
discontinuation of treatment

Your red blood cells which carry oxygen from your lungs to all of your cells are affected by the Ribavirin. The severity is quite individual. The red blood cells could break down at an abnormal rate or your bone marrow will not produce enough. At a minimum, you should have your hemoglobin checked at 2, 4, 8, and 12 wks after starting. Continue to have it checked every 4 wks after that. If you develop these symptoms, do not hesitate to call your health care provider and have your blood count checked. There are interventions which can be done, depending on your particular situation. If your hemoglobin drops below 10, your provider may suggest reducing your dose of Ribavirin or adding a drug (Procrit, epogen, Eprex) which stimulates your red cell production. Be prepared to have this discussion with your provider and ask about the pro and cons of both options.

Neutropenia

Interferon can contribute to bone marrow suppression of neutrophils and lymphocytes (white blood cells). This can interfere with a person's ability to fight infection. Frequently this occurs in the early weeks of treatment and then stabilizes. If it does not stabilize, dose reduction is a common strategy or the provider may decide to add a drug used to increase white blood cell and neutrophil counts. These blood counts should return to normal after treatment completion.

Thyroid

The thyroid gland can be affected by interferon. It can become overactive or under active. If you have ever had thyroid problems in the past, inform your health care provider. The thyroid is also monitored by a simple blood draw. An under active thyroid can cause hair to fall out, become dry, and become brittle, cause fatigue, and cause the skin to become dry. If a person feels like that already, an under-functioning thyroid may worsen those symptoms. It is very simple to manage an under active thyroid by taking medication daily. However, there is no guarantee that the thyroid will return to normal upon treatment completion. In that case, a person would have to continue on thyroid replacement with periodic monitoring of blood levels. Discuss any concerns you have about this with your health care provider.

Adverse side effects of HCV treatment can be managed. Talk to your provider honestly and often. Research is being done on new treatment medications, potentially decreasing some of the side effects currently experienced by patients undergoing HCV treatment with the current standard of care medications, Pegylated Interferon and Ribavirin. The goals of new research is to achieve a more rapid viral response while decreasing treatment time, reduce time spent managing medication side effects, and improve the HCV patient's quality of life.

Section References

1. Ong, J.P, & Younossi, Z.M. (May 2004). Cleveland clinic Journal of Medicine, vol.71, supplement 3.

2. Hepatitis C Choices: 4th ed. St. John, T.M. & Sandt, L. Caring Ambassadors Program, 2008.

3. www.clevelandclinic.org, Managing Side Effects of Hepatitis C Treatment, The Cleveland Clinic, Department of Patient Education and Health Information, 2008.

4. www.hepatitis.va.gov, Clinical Manual: Interferon and Ribavirin Treatment Side Effects, United States Department of Veteran Affairs, 2008.

5. www.hepcawareness.net.au, Treatment Side Effects, Australian Hepatitis Council, 2008.

12

Tools and Resources

Insurance and Other Resources

For an up to date comprehensive list of resources including pharmaceutical resources, patient medication assistance programs, support organizations and foundations, prescription assistance, clinical trials information, and consumer & governmental agencies, please go to www.hcvshare.org where you will find organized tables of the most recent updated online links to these resources.

Log Drop Calculations

The medical community looks at response to treatment using logarithmic math. They like to talk in terms of "log drops", or "absolute log values." You may have heard your doctor say something like, "We need to see at least a 2 log drop by week 12 of treatment for us to determine that you are responding to treatment." Indeed under normal standard of care (for Genotype 1 and 4), this is a required response to continue treatment. In the simplest terms, a 2 log drop is simply the point at which your viral load concentration has decreased to 1/100 of its starting, or baseline, concentration level; so, if your baseline concentration was 5,000,000 then a 2 log drop is when your concentration has dropped down to 50,000., or when a starting viral load of 1,000,000 had dropped to 10,000. Each 1 log drop is equal to a 9/10 (or 90%) drop.

Most people who have studied logarithms did so in algebra classes, and the majority has probably long forgotten what logarithms are all about. So, in this section, we will try to present a refresher for those who once studied logarithms and a mini-tutorial for those new to the concepts of logs. If you ever studied exponents and powers of 10, then you know $10^1 = 10$, $10^2 = 100$, $10^3 = 1000$. If you decrease your baseline viral load by a power of 10, you have gone down to 1/10 (one-tenth) of the baseline; for instance going from 1,000,000 to 100,000 is equal to a one log drop (one power of 10). If you drop to 1/100 (one-hundredth) of the baseline; for instance from 1,000,000 to 10,000, then that is a two log drop (two powers of 10).

Now, let's say we want to figure out what our viral load concentration would need to be for us to have achieved a 2 log drop if our starting viral load is 4,340,000. We simply need to divide that number by 2 powers of 10, or 100 to find out. So, to find the answer, we simply drop off the last 2 zeros in the number, and end up with 43,400. So, to review, to find out what the 2 log drop for a starting viral load is, just divide by 100. Now what if you want to track how you are doing along the way? That is a bit more challenging, but not too much, if one has a calculator or is familiar with using a spreadsheet application.

To calculate a particular log drop(ld) for a starting viral load (svl) and an ending viral load (evl), the formula to use is: $ld = LOG_{10}(evl/svl)$. For example, let's assume we have n svl of 1,000,000 and an evl of 10,000. Using the formula, the log drop (ld) = LOG_{10} (10,000/1,000,000) = -2, which means there was a 2 log drop (the negative sign, '-', indicates a drop, while a positive sign would indicate a rise in viral load). Now, we probably could have done that one in our head, because we know there were 2 powers of 10 drop. But for more obscure values, the formula comes in handy. In an a spreadsheet "cell" one would type in, "=LOG(evl/svl, 10)", where evl and svl are the end and starting viral load values, and the "10" represents the logarithm to the base 10. On a regular standard calculator, just punch in: evl / svl LOG. On an RPN style calculator, such as Hewlett Packard Brands, puch in: evl Enter svl / LOG.

SVR Estimator

At the outset here, let me say a few things about the process of attempting to calculate what the chances are one has for achieving a sustained viral response (SVR). First off, when one reads about chances for SVR in relation to say viral kinetics and ones own particular viral response to treatment, the value reported is based on statistical sampling. That's why the number is reported as a percentage. For instance, if the chances are reported as say 90% from a particular study for patients who achieved a rapid viral response (RVR), then what that means is that if 100 people who have the same characteristics as the people from the study achieve an RVR viral response, there is an expectation that 90 of those 100 people would achieve an SVR given the same circumstances under which the study was performed.

With that in mind, we can look at statistical responses to treatment in correlation with viral responses and come to some conclusions about what the expectation might be for an individual in terms of their chances for achieving SVR status based on their individual viral response to treatment in comparison to those from reported study results. Now again, the result we will come to will only be an approximate statistical representation, but will not be conclusive in any manner as to any one single individual, except in reference to expectations of a group to which that individual might belong.

Now, if the result for a particular analysis based on certain study results is, say 30% chance for SVR, that doesn't mean you, as an individual, should expect not to achieve an SVR, because you could easily belong to the 30% group. How the individuals who are in the 30% group differ from those in the 70% group is usually not always clear and represented. So, we should view particular statistical calculated percentages as relative indicators of likelihood predictors, giving us a sense of where we stand. For instance it is usually the case that those who clear the virus more quickly than others usually have a better chance of success as those who clear the virus later on in treatment, for a particular genotype, such as genotype 1.

With the background in mind, let's get on with the statistical and mathematical modeling of predicting then, where we stand based on when we first achieved an undetectable status, assuming in this example we are genotype 1. From the final results of the "SUCCESS" study, complete early viral response (cEVR – Undetected virus by week 12) SVR rates were 79.5%, and for slow responders (not undetected until sometime between weeks 12 and 24) treated for 48 weeks, the SVR rate was 43.0%[1]. Slow responders achieve UND status somewhere between week 12 and 24, so, assuming a normal probability population distribution for all patients in that group, we should take the average of the weeks 12 and 24 for the 43.0%, or week 18.

This simply means that we are assuming the average week for slow responders to reach undetected status is between weeks 12 and 24; it should be noted that this may have not been the case, but for this example, we are making this assumption. Similarly, assuming an average for cEVR, we will assume the average week that undetected status was achieved is between weeks 0 and 12, or week 6. Using these two data points, we can model the data assuming a linear relationship, which is appropriate for using first order Newtonian approximations. Using the linear equation based on the model, we can then plug in any week for first becoming undetected status and approximate the chances for SVR based on a statistical distribution of members falling within that group.

Now again, we must caution that this is in no way meant to be construed as an absolute prediction for any one particular individual, including you. There are individual circumstances that can come into play that will affect a particular person's outcome. For instance, some individuals have more advanced degree of liver damage than others and some have other more pronounced negative pretreatment indicators than others. But plugging in different weeks, should give us an indication of how ones chances of success changes with how early or late one clears the virus.

Here are the data points we use for our simple model:
UND week 6, SVR = 79.5%
UND week 18, SVR = 43.0%
If we interpolate by fitting a line to the two known data points, we will find that the SVR predicted rate (pr) for UND status at week X, is modeled by the equation:

pr= -3.0417*X+97.75.

Section References

1. M Buti, Y Lurie, NG Zakharova, and others. Extended treatment duration in chronic Hepatitis C genotype 1-infected slow responders: final results of the SUCCESS study. 44th Annual Meeting of the European Association for the Study of the Liver (EASL 2009). Copenhagen, Denmark. April 22-26, 2009.

Conclusions

In conclusion, HCV is a slow progressing disease. You will have time to learn much about it; the different treatment options that are available, and how to cope with the many different side effects brought on by the medications. Most experience many of the side effects, but many also manage to learn how to deal with them during the course of HCV treatment.

Your primary goal is to beat the virus while maintaining as healthy a lifestyle as possible. Keep aware of your side effects and keep your doctor informed of them all. Keep a list of questions as they arise and take them with you to your doctor visits. Remember to ask for a copy of all your lab work, so you will always have a record available.

Having a good support group to help you through this process is essential, whether they be composed of your family members, close friends, an online support forum, or combination of all of them. There will be times, when the available support will be a much needed relief to help you through some rough times that might arise.

Our greatest hope is that we have provided you with some information, experiences, and knowledge that help gives you the confidence, motivation, and tools necessary to improve your chances of conquering the Hepatitis C virus while surviving the treatment process. Our very best hope and prayers are with you.

About the Authors

Tim Duncan is an Engineering Manager educated in Physics with graduate level coursework in Statistical Process Analysis. He is husband to a loving wife and father of two wonderful children. Tim was diagnosed with HCV 6 years previous to going through treatment. He entered into a clinical trial in late 2009 and completed treatment in March 2010. During treatment, he met Catherine on an online HCV support network; he and Catherine subsequently entered into a collaboration to bring their research results, new found knowledge, and experiences to light in this guide.

Catherine Olivolo is a Family Nurse Practitioner, respected community leader, wife, mom and Noni to seven blessed grandchildren. She was diagnosed with the Hepatitis C virus in early 2009. At the time of this writing, she is still currently in treatment with an undetectable viral load. Her decision to collaborate on this book emphasizes her strong belief that anyone with HCV should have available accurate, essential information to increase the odds as much as possible for a successful HCV treatment outcome: SVR

Personal Notes

_____

_____

_____

_____

_____

_____

_____

_____

_____

Personal Notes

Personal Notes

Personal Notes

Personal Notes

Personal Notes

Personal Notes

Personal Notes

Personal Notes

Personal Notes

Personal Notes